PEACE

in the

STORM

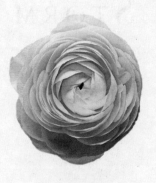

MAUREEN PRATT

PEACE
in the
STORM

MEDITATIONS
ON CHRONIC PAIN
AND ILLNESS

GALILEE | DOUBLEDAY
New York London Toronto Sydney Auckland

A GALILEE BOOK
PUBLISHED BY DOUBLEDAY
a division of Random House, Inc.

GALILEE and DOUBLEDAY are registered trademarks of
Random House, Inc., and the portrayal of a ship with a cross above a
book is a trademark of Random House, Inc.

First Galilee edition published May 2005

Book design by Nicola Ferguson

Library of Congress Cataloging-in-Publication Data
Pratt, Maureen.
    Peace in the storm : meditations on chronic pain and
illness / by Maureen Pratt.
        p. cm.
    Includes bibliographical references.
    1. Chronically ill—Prayer-books and devotions—English.
    2. Chronic pain—Patients—Prayer-books and devotions—English.
    I. Title.
BV4910.P73 2005
242'.4—dc22   2004056175

ISBN 0-385-51079-9

*To Jane Jordan Browne—mentor, agent,
fellow prayer warrior . . . friend*

The human spirit can endure a sick body,
but who can bear it if the spirit is crushed?

—*Proverbs 18:14, New Living Translation*

CONTENTS

Contents

Contents

xi

Contents

Contents

ACKNOWLEDGMENTS

There are many people I have to thank, but first I have to say that I am so grateful to the Lord for this opportunity, and I lift up to him all my song and praise.

Next, I would also like to thank my mother, for her never-ending support, love, and laughter. What a glorious gift God has given me in you!

My gratitude goes to Michelle Rapkin, my editor, for her guidance, insight, and humor. And to the rest of the team at Doubleday Religion—thank you, too!

To Danielle Egan-Miller, Cassie, Joanna, and all the great people at Browne & Miller Literary, I admire you and am delighted to be working with you. In memory of my late agent, Jane Jordan Browne, I praise God for letting me learn from the best.

Several people read parts of the early drafts of this book. To Cyndee, Katrina, Frank, Donie, Nancy, and Linda—thank you for your spirit, faith, and great suggestions!

My early writing years were deeply inspired by Walter J. Burghardt, S.J., and I would like to thank him for his encouragement and ever-continuing fellowship.

And to my fellow prayer warriors, "lupies," "fibros," hypothyroid sufferers, and everyone who also walks this path of illness and discovery, I give my prayers and encouragement—a stronger, more resilient group of remarkable men and women cannot be found!

Praise God for all of his many miraculous blessings!

INTRODUCTION

Living with a chronic illness is never easy, but I cannot imagine walking this road without the Lord. To be sure, there are times when pain overtakes any effort of mine to focus on prayer. And there are times when the days and nights seem so endlessly full of physical challenge that I am weary, truly weary, of even lifting a hand to read from the Word. Still, the only way for me to continue on in joy, hope, and faith is to believe, to know, that Jesus is right beside me each step, no matter how painful.

SICKNESS AND HEALTH . . .

My childhood was fraught with illness. By the time I was eighteen years old I had had pneumonia thirteen times, bronchitis, asthma, colitis, measles, mumps, chicken pox, and "basic" adolescence. I had been declared "terminal" by healthcare professionals on more than one occasion and had received the Sacrament of Last Rites. Still, as horrible as my illnesses seemed to be, and as endless, I recovered. After graduating from high school on time, I went away to college, earned my degree, and worked in high-profile, difficult jobs. I was a National Park Service "ranger" at the Lincoln Home and at the Kennedy Center. I worked in multilingual positions in Washington, D.C. I began working on a graduate degree at Carnegie Mellon University.

And I was diagnosed with Graves' disease.

The diagnosis derailed my grad school plans. I underwent treatment while working at international organizations. I felt better and moved on to a position as an MBA recruiter for a consulting firm, traveling across the country to campuses such as Harvard, Stanford, Wharton, and the University of Chicago. I completed translation course work and put my skills to use as a freelance translator, then applied once again to graduate schools and decided to attend UCLA's School of Theater, Film and Television. After earning my degree, I used my business and music skills, working in an office and conducting a church gospel choir. I assumed I would be working for a long time, building the choir, building a career. And then . . .

I was diagnosed with a severe case of lupus.

Then Sjogren's Syndrome, Hashimoto's thyroiditis, vasculitis, and fibromyalgia.

My whole world and expectations turned upside down. It was as if the Lord was crafting two people of me—the one who was productive and the one who was sick! How could I make sense of this duality? How could I continue to live, be productive, and witness as my body was wracked with challenge after challenge, pain upon pain?

The answer to these questions could not readily be found in the world around me. Illness, especially one that is severe and/or chronic, is often construed as weakness. Missing days of work, being unable to keep social commitments, going from one health crisis to another—all of these take the sufferer away from the conventional world and the people who move about in it. People who can't "keep up" are often dismissed or discarded—by friends, colleagues, even family members. Mis-information about chronic illnesses can circulate, making the sufferer a kind of pariah, much like the lepers in the Bible.

Also, because many illnesses are "incurable," the medical community can often dismiss a sufferer, saying, "There's really nothing we can do."

"Live with it," they might tell the patient.

To which we sufferers reply, "That's easy to say. But how do we really do that?"

A FIRM FOUNDATION

Throughout my youth and young adulthood, I was a believer. I read the Bible cover to cover, soaking up every word, every story of God's loving power and saving grace. I found hope there, and grace. I found examples in Job, Mary, and Jesus that gave me role models for handling my own difficulties. The simplicity and beauty of Psalms, Corinthians, and Proverbs lifted my heart and gave me sustenance for my journey.

But it wasn't until I was diagnosed with lupus and my struggle with serious illness reached a new height that I truly began to understand how remarkable, how crucial the peace of Christ is in the midst of the "storm"—the battle for health of spirit.

Lupus has no medical cure. In lupus, one's own body produces antibodies that attack internal organs and tissues, causing excruciating inflammation and complications that, at their "mildest," result in pain and bone-numbing fatigue and, at their worst, result in failure of organ systems (kidneys perhaps, or lungs). Some lupus patients die from complications stemming from the disease, long-term medication side effects, or other lupus-related problems.

Truly, the diagnosis of lupus sent me smack into the midst

of a raging, out-of-control storm. I had to stop working, personal relationships fell apart, my body was at war with itself. There were some days (and still are) when I could not get out of bed. Medications designed to combat symptoms caused bad side effects. Performing simple tasks, such as cooking or doing the laundry, seemed monumental and often impossible.

Turning again to Scripture, I had new questions, fervent questions. My prayer life became a kind of constant search for meaning, strength, and calm.

And through this initial reaction to the diagnosis and knowledge that I'd probably be living with lupus awhile, the Lord responded. He worked to give me the right doctors, the right sense of humor. He knew I needed a lot of time to rest and sleep, and he gave that to me. And, as always in the past, he has been with me each step of the way.

He answers my cries and my prayers with profound, lasting peace.

The search for this peace has brought me closer than ever to Scripture and the Lord. It has also moved me closer to a faith community that encompasses not only my home church, but Christians the world over who also struggle with illness. We encourage one another, we laugh and cry with one another. We marvel at the peace that comes only from communion with Christ.

How does one reach this peace? And how does one keep hold of it?

MAKING SENSE, MAKING PEACE

In order to reach peace and maintain it, we have to realize our humanness. We have to admit we suffer from pain, sorrow, guilt, loneliness . . . all of the many emotions that can weigh us down. We also have to acknowledge that there is joy in our suffering, and hope. We can find laughter in life, and triumph over even the slightest of difficulties. If we recognize our emotions and are able to articulate what we are going through, we can lift up prayers that address these things specifically. We can take our illness piece by piece, lift it all up to the Lord—and not have to take it back again!

Like our Lord in the garden on the night he was betrayed, after we have acknowledged our deep humanity, we can turn to God and say, "Thy will be done."

And then we shall feel a quiet, a peace that transcends all suffering and all pain.

This is not to say that we will be physically cured. Sometimes this is the Lord's will and sometimes it is not, and no amount of petitioning or expectation will make us change the Lord's will. But it is to say that we will have healthy spirits, healthy inner lives. And this attention to spiritual well-being can make a tremendous difference in our overall health, our entire outlook on the world, and our place in it.

FOUR "HARBORS"

There are four "harbors" to anchor the spirit in the quest to finding peace in the storm:

- Recognizing the changeable nature of illness (you *know* some days are better than others) and acknowledging the constant nature of the Lord (he is *always* with you, even when you're not thinking of him);
- Taking time out from your day to have true quiet time in prayer and in listening to the Lord;
- Taking the bad with the good that can come from living with illness and celebrating these good things as gifts and joys;

- Nurturing relationships—having friends and being a friend to others.

The Nature of Chronic Pain and Illness

The word "chronic" means "ongoing." A chronic illness or pain will be with you for a long time—possibly the rest of your earthly life. But your medical condition will not necessarily be constant in intensity, symptoms, or severity. Some days, your pain will be horrible. Other days, you will have relief. Your illness might be unpredictable; perhaps you have lupus and never quite know what the next day will bring. Or your illness might be more foreseeable; perhaps your arthritis is worse only if there is a rainstorm on the horizon. If you are a cancer patient undergoing chemotherapy, you will certainly experience swings in how you feel and how much energy you have, depending on where you are in your treatment.

Coping with the ups and downs of chronic illness and/or pain is one of the most difficult aspects of this life. It is also one of the most difficult things for healthy people to understand. But, as with everything, the Lord understands.

"Don't you know that the Lord is the everlasting God, the Creator of all the earth? He never grows faint or weary. No one can measure the depths of his understanding. He gives power to those who are tired and worn out; he offers strength to the weak. Even youths will become exhausted, and young men will give up. But those who wait on the Lord will find new strength. They will fly high on wings like eagles. They will run and not grow weary. They will walk and not faint."
—*Isaiah 40:28–31, New Living Translation*

Think about this passage. Read it over several times. Take it into your heart, pondering the greatness of the Lord. He *knows* you may be exhausted, ready to throw in the towel. But wait. Wait for the next day. Wait for the pain to subside. Give yourself and your body time. Even against the ever-changing, heart-wrenching landscape of living with chronic illness, the Lord is there, ready to give you new strength, new hope.

He is *always* with you.

BEING TRULY STILL

Finding the peace of the Lord within requires taking time to be truly and completely still. This means that you open your ears and heart only to the Lord, shutting out all distractions, including those of your own petitions and desires. In fact, your only desire to seeking peace should be to hear the Lord's voice—in Scripture and in your heart. This might seem like an impossible task. But Jesus, awaiting his arrest and crucifixion, sets the example.

"Your will be done."
—*Matthew 26:42, New American Bible*

Take time each day to sit in as comfortable a position as possible so you won't be distracted by pain. Shut your ears to even the slightest noise. Close your eyes so they don't wander over the objects around you. Begin with one of the prayers or meditations in this book, so you can focus on the Lord. And then listen. Listen to the whisper of his word. Remember, he is always present, and he is ready to give you what you need when you need it.

In the stillness, in the quiet, you will draw nearer to him.

And this quiet, this peace, will strengthen you, even in the most awful of times.

SERIOUS ILLNESS CAN BE POSITIVE?!

Living with a serious illness sets you apart from many other people, and often this is a difficult, sad thing. But through your trials, you will find strength, resilience, creativity, and insight that others who are healthy do not usually encounter. Living with illness makes you the toughest of survivors. It makes you more aware of triumphs, great and small. It gives you a greater appreciation for life, relationships, faith, and growth.

Think of how much you have to offer others! You can minister to people who are afraid of illness or pain, who doubt the Lord's presence in their lives. You can reflect the joy of God's creation even more strongly because some days all you can do is watch the birds fly and the breeze blow in the world around you. How many other people, healthy people, do this often enough to be filled with awe and reverence? Not many. But you can. You do.

By taking proper care of your body, you demonstrate to others the importance of respecting God's creation of you. What a witness you can be to people who might be tempted to experiment with drugs, to those who smoke, drink excessively, or abuse their bodies in other ways. What a loving testimony to God's presence on earth!

Yes, there are many benefits to having a chronic medical condition. And in this sense, your illness or pain is a gift. Thinking positively about it and finding ways to use it to God's greater glory are giant steps toward coming to terms with it—and to finding peace.

WE ARE EVANGELISTS

Christians who suffer from illness and pain need not, in fact, *should* not, be cut off from the world.

> "You are the light of the world—like a city on a mountain, glowing in the night for all to see. Don't hide your light under a basket! Instead, put it on a stand and let it shine for all."
> —*Matthew 5:14–15, New Living Translation*

You?

Yes, you!

Don't wait for a cure to make friends, witness to others, lend a helping hand to those in need. Don't hide the story of God's work in your life, of the way he brings you strength, hope, and comfort. Having friends and being a friend to others is essential to allowing the Lord to work. So, assess what you can do, be positive about developing nurturing relationships, and go! Remember, the Lord will be with you all along the way.

WHAT ABOUT THIS BOOK?

Each of the above four "harbors" will be covered in many ways throughout the rest of this book. There are thoughts and images to reflect upon and prayers to help you form petitions and articulate aspects of your illness. There is blank space on which you can write your own thoughts and reactions to the material here. And there are practical ways to help you reach out to others in faith communities and beyond.

Instead of being a day-to-day sort of guide, this book addresses many different aspects of living with chronic pain and illness. These include sorrow, loneliness, hope, fatigue, and faith. It is up to you whether you take the book page-by-page or dip into it as you feel the need. There is no right or wrong way to use this book—the important thing is that you use it.

YOU ARE UNIQUE AND LOVED

Sometimes, when we live with an illness and in pain, we begin to think that our identity is that of the medical condition. You might think of yourself as a "diabetic" or a "cancer patient." But this is only one part of who you are. As the saying goes, we are each as different as snowflakes. Finding peace within will help you rediscover aspects of yourself that have been overwhelmed by your illness. You will also begin to explore other gifts that the Lord will give you as you become stronger and more determined to have a full, productive, and joyful life.

Each step of your journey through pain to calm, setback to triumph, will demonstrate all the more definitively that you *are* more than your illness. You *are* unique and special. You have much to be thankful for. Much to give.

And you are loved. Completely. In spite of your illness. Forever.

You are loved by the Lord.

PEACE
in the
STORM

WHY ME?

"You are my witnesses," declares the Lord,
"And my servant whom I have chosen,
so that you may know and believe me and understand that I am he.
Before me no god was formed, nor will there be one after me.
I, even I, am the Lord, and apart from me there is no savior.
I have revealed and saved and proclaimed—
I and not some foreign god among you.
You are my witnesses," declares the Lord, "That I am God."
—Isaiah 43:10–12, New International Version

The first days and weeks after being diagnosed with a serious, chronic medical condition are full of questions. Indeed, it is almost as if we have become children again, having to learn how to live by a new set of rules and how to exist in a new and frightening world. This parallel continues to the questions we ask, chief among them, "Why?" We try to think of whom or what we might have come into contact with that would have infected us, or what mix of genes and environmental factors combined to bring about our illness. Was it something we ate? Something we did? Something someone else said, did, or didn't do? We comb through medical information, looking for answers. And we lift our queries to the heavens, asking God, as our Father, the same question we

posed to our parents who told us to do things we didn't want
to do (like chores, or sharing a toy).

"Why me?"

Now, in our seeming adulthood, we probably add many
more words to this question when we direct it to the Lord:

"Of all the people on the face of the earth, why did this illness strike me? Surely others are less diligent about keeping
healthy. Surely others have more time to be ill. What about my
faithful following of your teachings, Lord? Doesn't my belief
in you give me an edge over those who have fallen away or,
worse, have refused to listen to you? And, if you had to bring
illness into my life, why did you give me something so terrible? A cold, a few headaches, the gentle physical manifestations of growing a bit older—these I would have borne in
relative ease. But this? My Lord, because of this illness, my life
has been turned upside down. Oh, it's true that I haven't been
feeling well for a while. But my plans for the future, my careful financial planning, my close relationships are all affected by
my malady. And for what purpose? Truly, before this illness,
my life was going along so well! Why me?"

We wait for a response from the Lord, but his answer
eludes us. So, we keep asking, just as we did when we were
children. But remember what our parents used to say in response to our questioning their requests? It might even be
what you say to your children under the same circumstances.
Certainly, it's the answer that God provides us with now.

"Because I said so."

Indeed, God does not have to reveal his reasons for drawing us down the path we're on. At least, not yet. He is omnip-
otent, over all things, including ourselves. He is the ultimate
parent, his way *is* the highway. And he wants us to allow him
to lead. The more time we spend questioning his motives, the
less time we will have for embracing the experiences and in-
sights reserved for us by the Lord.

In this reading from Isaiah, God says he has chosen us to be his witnesses. How wonderful that we are chosen by him, loved by him for our whole lives! His special witnesses, in spite of, along with, our life-altering illness. Can we, then, mistrust him? Question the way he is working in our lives?

Surely not!

Anything that comes from God is good. And by our faith, our trust in him, our triumphs over adversity, and our love, we are living proof of this.

Father in heaven, you know the questions that weigh heavily upon my heart.
Just as I rejoice that you have chosen me to be witness to your awesome might,
help me move from childhood to maturity about my illness.
Let me not resist your plan for me, but go willingly, proclaiming to all that you are God.

ACCEPTING YOUR DIAGNOSIS

For sighing comes more readily to me than food,
and my groans well forth like water.
For what I fear overtakes me,
and what I shrink from comes upon me.
I have no peace nor ease;
I have no rest, for trouble comes!
—Job 3:24–26, New American Bible

Accepting a diagnosis of serious illness is like peeling a pungent onion. Even as we take off the layers of doubt, disbelief, and refusal to accept, our eyes well up with tears and our fingers tremble. The onion is an unsettling element, being added with much discomfort to the stew of other ingredients that make up our lives. The task becomes exceedingly painful, even excruciating, the longer we peel back the layers and drop them into the mix. We'd rather do without it. But at this moment, our life's recipe calls for a complete onion, and we must continue. When we reach the onion's core, finally, we are able to dry our tears and turn to the meal at hand. So, too, after we can fully accept our diagnosis, we can cleanse our hearts for the time that lies ahead—the time of tasting the onion-flavored "stew" and benefiting fully from the new and more healthful concoction that will nourish us in the days and years ahead.

Before I was diagnosed with lupus, I held the firm belief

that whatever was wrong could be dealt with quickly and effectively. I remember facing one doctor and saying, "So, you'll give me some medication and I'll be fine, right?" I truly had no idea how serious lupus was, nor did I fully realize what the diagnosis would mean to all aspects of my life. Looking back on those first few weeks of coping with all the information I learned about lupus, as well as the seemingly endless (and often painful) tests I had to undergo and the medications I had to purchase and start taking, I realize that I didn't *want* to "fully realize" everything all at once.

Indeed, accepting my diagnosis of lupus took a long time. During that period, I did a lot of sighing and groaning as I adjusted the many facets of my life to accommodate the changes lupus brought to them. When I could no longer hide my hair loss, I bought a wig, threw it on the floor in disgust when I couldn't immediately fit it on my head without thinking it looked fake—and picked it up, brushed it off, and tried again. I insisted upon pushing through excruciating lupus fatigue in an effort to somehow prove that it could be conquered—and discovered it could not. I told people I was "fine" when I really wasn't—and felt resentment when they weren't as sympathetic as I thought they should have been.

During this journey with lupus, I have learned that some amount of denial can be surprisingly healthy in the immediate wake of a diagnosis. If we accepted the complete scope of serious illness all at once, we might fall into a shock so profound that we'd be unable to move along toward a more healthful life. So, instead of being overwhelmed, we peel back the onion, feeling the sting of the tears as we do so, and accept our diagnosis piece by piece until we are able to accept it all—and be the better for it.

O Lord, please help me in my unbelief.
As I work through the reality of the illness from which
I suffer,

let me be ever mindful of your hand upon me.
Let me see the truth of my life and accept what you have
given me,
so that I may make the most of all,
for the continued strength of my body and soul
and the glory of your name.

LONELINESS

Do not be afraid or discouraged, for the Lord is the one who goes before you. He will be with you; he will neither fail nor forsake you.

—*Deuteronomy 31:8, New Living Translation*

I magine you are hiking with three of your loved ones in a dense mountain forest. The trees—birch, pine, and oak—are so thick and rise so far above your head that they obscure the far-off sun. Beneath your feet, the uneven ground is strewn with rocks, withered pine cones, and thick tree roots as it spirals upward, making your way dangerous, even though the path is well defined. Here and there are marvels of God's handiwork: a waterfall cascading down an embankment and into a rippling river, a delicate eggshell blue wildflower peeping out of the crevice of a rotten log. There are forest birds, too, whose songs fill the air with shrill music. And beyond all this, at the end of the path, you are sure there will be something even more marvelous than this gentle unfolding of nature.

Suddenly, midway up a steep part of the path, you hear a sharp crack. Three forest birds streak across your view and away from the disturbance. You think of mad dogs, bears, and wolves. Your heart fills with fear. But before you can reach out to your companions for safety, two of your loved ones run away, disappearing rapidly down the path, and the third scoots up a nearby tree. In moments you are standing alone, with the sound of something terrible getting closer with each passing second.

The feeling of utter loneliness is a bitter, fearful sensation that there is no one to turn to, no one to be with you at your time of need. When you were diagnosed with your illness, you might have experienced this. Perhaps a trusted loved one didn't believe your diagnosis or accused you of doing something to bring it on. You feel a rift now, at a time when you most need the comfort and safety of a friend.

After your diagnosis, you continue to experience loneliness. People you thought were friends move away from you, especially as your illness makes it more difficult for you to be energetic and sociable. Your spouse becomes physically and emotionally distant; as your body changes and the illness affects your appearance and personality, he or she might even begin to wonder if the marriage will stay together. This insecurity about your future, even if you took vows of "for better, for worse," can be terrifying. Not only do you feel lonely in the moment, you fear a future of a marriage promise broken, a trust betrayed.

Loved ones are not the only ones who might move away from you. Coworkers resent your illness because they have to do your work as well as theirs when you can't be productive. They separate themselves from you and you become isolated at work.

Some animals prey on the weakest among them; it seems as though some people want to figuratively treat you that way, too. From insurance battles to getting the wheelchair to come to the airport gate when you arrive, you always seem to be alone and vulnerable. In your illness, pain, and fear, you feel more than loneliness. You feel desolation.

On the mountain forest path, alone and afraid, you are angry that your friends have deserted you. But do you allow your mind to go blank from fear, anger, and resentment?

At this very harrowing crossroads, you have a choice to make. If you want to continue in stark loneliness, you will continue to dwell on it, let it chase you down and tear you apart. But if you want to forge your courage in the face of adversity and rise above despair to someplace better, you need to call upon something deeper and closer to your heart and soul than your very human loneliness.

You need to call upon the Lord.

Look inward and breathe deeply. Ask for strength.

"Do not be afraid or discouraged, for the Lord is the one who goes before you. He will be with you; he will neither fail nor forsake you."

The Lord is more powerful than all our fears combined. He created you and me. He is with us through everything, through every step on our journey to the summit of the mountain.

Out of human fear, your loved ones have run from the unseen peril that is closing in. You cannot run from it, but you can face it with the courage that comes from belief in the presence of God in your life. By your courage, you will show your loved ones and everyone you meet that you have no intention of letting your illness separate you from the creation God has made and from your beloved friends, family members, and colleagues.

Staring down the monster, you intimidate it and it slinks back into the forest. You shout for your loved one to come down from the tree. You reach out to the other two companions who have run away. You tell them, "It's all right. We'll be safe. Come, let's continue on."

And so, you do. Soon the forest gives way to a smooth slab of granite forged from centuries of upheaval and weathering. The view is spectacular! Miles and miles of glorious azure sky and brilliant sun, deep green trees and glittering waterways. It is the earth. It is life. It is peace. And you made it here because you trusted in God to take away your fear, your loneliness.

He has given you this wondrous gift of living to enjoy in spite of your illness.

By his grace, you do. And, best of all, you share it with your loved ones.

> *Lord, there is an emptiness in me that cries out for you.*
> *There are feelings within me of utter loneliness,*
> *as if the whole world has abandoned me.*
> *Take away my despair and let me feel your comforting*
> *hand upon me.*
> *For you are my Lord and Savior and you are my*
> *best friend.*
> *Now and always.*

WHEN THE "YOU" YOU KNEW
SEEMS TO DISAPPEAR

"Remember not the events of the past,
the things of long ago consider not;
See, I am doing something new!
Now it springs forth, do you not perceive it?
In the desert, I make a way,
in the wasteland, rivers."
—*Isaiah 43:18–19, New American Bible*

"I used to be thinner."
"My hair used to be light blond."
"I could run miles and not get tired."
"I never used to be this forgetful."
"I hardly know myself anymore."

The "you" before you became sick and the "you" now are probably very different from one another. Serious illness and pain can change our bodies, minds, and abilities. Indeed, the whole world in which we live can become completely different. Instead of pickup basketball games or movie dates, you might be filling your schedule with doctor visits, dialysis, chemotherapy, and radiation treatments. Restful nights might be replaced by pain-filled darkness. Stalwart independence might give way to a childlike reliance on others.

As the days go by and we leave more of our healthy days behind, it is natural to yearn more and more for those happier times. Looking at old photographs might bring up memories of how much better you thought you looked before your illness robbed you of your healthy skin and hair. Athletic equipment gathering dust in a closet might remind you of the activity you used to enjoy and the people with whom you used to enjoy it. You might feel as though you're suspended in a kind of nightmare of illness. You mourn your loss, feeling it so profoundly that you cry.

Where *is* the "you" you used to know?

Will you ever be the way you once were?

As difficult as it is sometimes to take to heart, our lives do not end with the onset of a serious illness. Until the day we breathe our last earthly breath, life goes on and we continue to move forward, following in faith the Lord's path for us. We carry with us our memories of the past and we think on many of them fondly. But we cannot deny the present, nor can we ignore that the Lord continues to work in our lives throughout our illness and beyond.

"See, I am doing something new!
Now it springs forth, do you not perceive it?"

The Lord promises he will make a way in the desert, "in the wasteland, rivers." He will do the same in our lives. If we cling to the past and stay mired in our memories, we won't experience the promises the Lord makes. But if we allow him to work his "something new" in us, we will fully benefit from his way, his promise fulfilled.

O Lord, I cry when I think of the strength and health
I used to enjoy.
I miss the days of happiness and pleasure, the things
and people who filled my hours.

But I know, Lord, that you are still with me,
leading me and guiding me.
And I ask that, even as I treasure my memories,
you help me welcome the goodness that you bring
from now on.

You Are Being Refined

But who can endure the day of his coming? Who can stand when he appears? For he will be like a refiner's fire or a launderer's soap. He will sit as a refiner and purifier of silver; he will purify the Levites and refine them like gold and silver. Then the Lord will have men who will bring offerings in righteousness, and the offerings of Judah and Jerusalem will be acceptable to the Lord, as in the days gone by, as in former years.

—Malachi 3:2–4, New International Version

Before they become gleaming jewels set in glittering gold, platinum, or silver, gemstones and precious metals must undergo a sometimes violent process of refinement. Wrested from the earth by means of digging, blasting, and painstaking physical effort, the substances are transported to places aboveground, then they are separated from their host rocks where they have resided for eons. The lot of resulting material is examined, sorted according to size and potential, and sold. Once again it is transported to workshops where more transformation occurs. Precious metals are purified—made molten so as to be broken down into their most basic form—then blended with other alloys to render them stronger and more resistant to scratching. The blend of metals is then molded, hammered, cut, heated, and treated with acids to be fashioned into forms that will eventually accept gemstones, becoming part of a whole.

Meantime, the gemstones are reexamined, marked, sawed, calibrated, etched, trimmed, polished, and perhaps treated with oils, colorings, heat, or radiation. They may become completely different in color and light refraction, almost unrecognizable compared to their original, raw appearance. Sometimes they crack or break completely from the pressure under which they are being refined. The craftspeople might even have to toss them aside if they are beyond repair.

Finally the gemstones and precious metals meet. Master jewelers and other craftspeople make from them objects of beauty to be enjoyed for generations—under the best of circumstances.

The Lord has already promised us that we are most precious to him. He wants us to be with him through eternity, so he puts us through "the fire," refining us and purifying us like the most valuable of gemstones or metals. Our purpose, our actions, might change as God develops us into the people we are meant to be. And he "treats" us through heat, pressure, and other metals to make us stronger, more righteous, more forceful in our obedience to him and more ready to be with him in heaven.

As one of the many challenges we have to face, our illness is but part of the process of lifelong refinement and purification. We go through ups and downs with it, and, with the Lord's craftsmanship, we become stronger and more courageous until finally we will be radiant as the most glittering diamond, ready to praise him throughout the rest of all eternity.

O Lord, sometimes I don't think I have the
strength to continue.

But help me to be willing, Lord, to allow you to use me
and fashion me,
according to your specifications.
For I know that through this refining and purification,
I will be made strong and be righteous,
worthy enough to stand in your presence forever.

YOUR BODY IS WONDERFUL

I give thanks, O Lord, with all my heart.
I will sing your praises before the gods.

* * *

You made all the delicate, inner parts of my body
and knit me together in my mother's womb.
Thank you for making me so wonderfully complex!
Your workmanship is marvelous—and how well I know it.
—Psalm 138:1; 139:13–14, New Living Translation

I am in awe of the creation that is the human body. It is so delicate and yet so strong. So simple and yet so complex. I am not aware of the beating of my heart, but it continues its work. I do not consciously tell my legs to move or my eyes to blink, and yet they do. When I think of all that my skin provides by way of protection, comfort, and beauty, I smile. When I think of all that goes on beneath my skin, I just shake my head in utter amazement. And when I think of the part the Lord as Creator has in all this, I tremble. For I cannot imagine the depth of the love he has for me, for you, to have given us such a wonderful gift! Yes, truly, our bodies are amazing.

But when something goes wrong, when we become ill, our perception of our bodies can change drastically. We may say our bodies have become "defective," "inferior," or even hateful to us. The failure of an organ, the withering of a limb, the malfunction of delicate nerve impulses—all of these can lessen our opinion of our bodies and lead us to criticize the very creation the Lord made *in his image.*

Outside influences can also contribute to a lesser opinion of our bodies. Advertisements that imply dissatisfaction with body image abound. Whole industries have sprung up to encourage "physical transformation" through elective plastic surgery or other cosmetic changes. We hear stories of athletes using artificial means to "bulk up" and of teenagers who succumb to anorexia or bulimia to maintain unhealthful (but perceived optimum) weight. Indeed, if we put all of these and other negative messages together, we might conclude that our bodies are inferior and that we each have to do something to improve upon them.

But, even if you are seriously ill, think of this:

In spite of all you are going through, your body *is* working.

With this in mind and heart, it becomes easier for each of us to appreciate and treasure our bodies and do what we can to healthfully enhance their function and appearance. A decorative hat, a new shirt, specially prepared meals, extra rest and comfort—all of these and more can help us move away from our criticism and toward love for God's gift to us.

Even though it might be less healthy than it could be, even though you must rely on extensive medical help, your body is still remarkable—and for that, all thanks and praise be to God our Father, who made us "so wonderfully complex."

O Lord, my God, I sometimes take for granted
the miraculous gift that is my body.
I am critical of its weaknesses and disdainful of its
shortcomings.
But in spite of my human disappointment, my body
continues to work!
Help me, Lord, to fully treasure and protect this
wondrous gift,
work of your hands and miracle of my life.

FINDING THE RIGHT DOCTOR

Cry out for insight and understanding.
Search for them as you would for lost money or hidden treasure.
Then you will understand what it means to fear the Lord,
And you will gain knowledge of God.
—*Proverbs 2:3–5, New Living Translation*

If you knew of a hidden treasure, you'd probably go to great lengths to find it. Besides following a map (if there were one), you'd keep your ears and eyes open for clues as to its whereabouts and brave any obstacle to get to it. Moreover, you'd follow your intuition, your "sense" of where the treasure might be. You might have to spend a lot of time looking and go out of your way to search. There might be dead ends and disappointments.

But you wouldn't give up until you held the treasure firmly in your hands.

The right doctor is certainly a treasure! Someone who is compassionate and competent, willing to communicate *and* listen, is to be valued, is worth looking for.

But how do you find such a person?

Not all physicians have the same training, and not all communicate in the same way even if they have the same background. Not all physicians make you comfortable with the level and kind of care you receive. Not all have experience with your illness.

But one of the doctors in this country—probably more than one—will give you the attention and treatment that you need.

Locating and identifying the right doctor takes work, but it also takes insight and understanding. True, you need to look at a physician's credentials, the parameters of your health plan, and your budget and location constraints. Personal recommendations are wonderful, as are doctor-to-doctor referrals. But even as important as all these search tools are, you need to lift up your search in prayer as you follow your good sense of what you need and desire.

As you try to discern who is right for you, look deep within you, quietly and completely. Face your prejudices and misgivings.

Do you think a particular doctor might be too old? Too young? Too black? Too white?

Do you think a male doctor is better than a female doctor?

Are you intimidated by a doctor who has high-level credentials?

Does a doctor's nationality put you off?

As you search through lists and make appointments, keep one finger on your own pulse of being comfortable, of being confident. Let God lead you away from your personal prejudices and toward the doctor who is just right for you.

Once you find the right doctor, treasure him or her! Be on time for appointments, be prepared with your lists of medications, symptoms, and questions.

Honor your doctor's time and attention.

And every now and then, tell your physician how much you appreciate the care you are receiving.

You deserve the best care possible. A good doctor deserves to be treasured.

PEACE IN THE STORM

O Lord, give me eyes to see and ears to hear clearly,
without prejudice,
who is the right doctor for me.
If I am not under that physician's care right now,
please lead me to him or her.
And help me to see ways to treasure that doctor,
just as much as you, my Heavenly Father, treasure me.

PRAYER FOR DOCTORS

"Then the king will say to those on the right, 'Come you who are blessed by my Father, inherit the Kingdom prepared for you from the foundation of the world. For I was hungry, and you fed me. I was thirsty, and you gave me a drink. I was a stranger, and you invited me into your home. I was naked, and you gave me clothing. I was sick, and you cared for me. I was in prison, and you visited me.'"

—*Matthew 25:34–36, New Living Translation*

A doctor dedicates a good part of his or her life to learning. Through college, medical school, residency, fellowships, and continuing education, a doctor acquires information that is, truly, astounding. But more important, a doctor puts all that learning to the practice of helping others.

Sometimes the doctor is on call all day and night. Often the doctor must perform procedures and operations that are gruesome, delicate, lifesaving. The doctor has to handle angry, desperate, sobbing, incredulous patients—and somehow overcome their emotions to help them understand their illness and treatment.

Think of your doctor and what he or she does in a day. Hospital rounds, consultations, follow-up appointments, new diagnoses, personal reading, journal-writing, record-keeping, prescription refills, emergency treatments. And then he or she tends to family, friends, and a personal life!

Doctors are often seen as superhuman and yet they are people, too. They have illnesses, doubts, fears, midlife crises, triumphs, and defeats.

How many people do you know, besides doctors, who attend to others at birth, in life, and at death?

With all that they do and all that they are, it is no wonder that good doctors will be at the Lord's right hand.

Do we also appreciate them?

If we have to wait for hours in the office before being seen, do we get aggravated?

If we expect them to cure us rapidly, do we think they're failing if they don't?

Do we think they are overpaid?

In every profession there are good and bad practitioners. Of course, we should be given the best care, the most respect, and not fall prey to greed. But if you think of the doctors who are involved with your care now, you will probably be amazed at how much they do for you and for others. There are probably many other professions they could have chosen, but medicine is their calling and they carry it out willingly, joyfully, compassionately.

Thinking of the good doctors you know, you will undoubtedly be struck with admiration.

These health warriors, these tireless caregivers, deserve our respect, earn our appreciation, and merit our heartfelt thanks and prayers.

O Lord, bless all doctors
with your comfort, strength, and wisdom.
Give them hope when they despair,

and faith when they are lost.
Bring them rest by night
and resilience by day.
Let them know that they are appreciated,
and that all their hard work is not in vain.

WHERE IS GOD?

My God, my God! Why have you forsaken me?
Why do you remain so distant?
Why do you ignore my cries for help?
Every day I call for you, my God, but you do not answer.
Every night you hear my voice, but I find no relief.
—Psalm 22:1–2, New Living Translation

Have you ever needed to speak with someone urgently, but couldn't reach him or her? Instead of being able to communicate directly, you end up leaving multiple messages. The first might be simple: "Please call me." The second might be more tentative: "I don't know if you got my first message, so I'm leaving this one." By the third call, your anxiety increases: "I hope you're all right . . . please call." By the fourth and subsequent times, you might also be irritated: "Where are you? Why haven't you called back? I need to speak with you or I wouldn't be calling." The longer your plea goes unanswered, the more persistent you might become, calling incessantly day *and* night.

Finally, weary from so much futile calling, you pause in the midst of dialing. And in the new-fallen silence, you hear a knock at the door. Puzzled, you go to the door and open it. Standing before you is the very person whom you were trying to reach by telephone.

"Why didn't you come to the door earlier?" the person asks. "I've been out here for hours, knocking, but you must not have heard me. Let me in. I think I have the answers you're looking for."

The simple answer to the question "Where is God?" is, "He is everywhere." But when we have a serious illness, the question takes on a very personal, urgent tone.

"Where is God in my life? In this suffering? In my ever-shrinking world?"

As we call upon God, sometimes we can't or don't feel his presence. Our pain is so acute that it interferes with our ability to sense him. Our minds are clouded by medication or worry. Indeed, our illness requires so much of our attention and energy that we might not hear even the most obvious manifestations of God's voice, of his answer to our prayers.

Deeply enmeshed in our own situation, we might doubt that God could be present in our suffering. If God wants the best for us, why would he take a personal part in bringing illness? We might expect that God would take away our suffering completely instead of letting it continue. As creatures of habit, too, we might look for the Lord in the same places we always have—in church, amidst our families, in fellowship—and be at a loss to find him in our new surroundings of medical facilities and sickrooms.

As our prayers to God become more strident and as our illness continues, we become more agitated. To the extreme, we equate God's hearing our prayers for help and health with his desire for the best for us, and we are wracked with disappointment when these prayers go seemingly unanswered. Our faith can be shaken to its core. We might stop praying altogether, stop raising our voices to the Lord. But when we finally allow ourselves to be quiet, to pause, to let our ears take over from our mouth, it is then that we experience the miracle. It is then that we hear God's voice.

It is almost impossible to hear someone else speak if we are talking all the time. But if we are silent, then we can hear. It is the same with our relationship with the Lord. He is present as we speak. He does hear us—all the time. We have only to let our ears take over in order to hear his response and feel his comfort, the comfort that he so dearly wishes to give us.

O Lord, I lift my voice to you, I cry to you day
and night.
But even before I do, you know what I am going to say.
You know how I feel. You know what I need.
Give me the strength and will to listen to you.
Quiet my tongue so that I may be fully in your presence
and hear your healing voice.

Finding Meaning in a
Life of Illness

Oh, the depth of the riches of wisdom and knowledge of God!
How inscrutable are his judgments and how unsearchable his ways!

"For who has known the mind of the Lord,
or who has been his counselor?
Or who has given him anything
that he may be repaid?"

For from him and through him and for him are all things. To him
be glory forever. Amen.
—*Romans 11:33–36, New American Bible*

W hat does it mean to be ill, to suffer from a serious sickness that might even threaten your life? Does it point
out a fundamental weakness within you or a personality flaw
that you failed to do something about sooner? Does it mean
that your life was headed in the wrong direction and the Lord
brought about your illness so that he could set you back on the
right track?

Can you figure out the connection between the kind of illness you have and the particular lesson you are supposed to
learn from it? If you have cancer, for example, what are you to
derive from the experience of surgery, chemotherapy, radiation

treatment, and long-term recovery? If you have rheumatoid arthritis, what does it mean that your body aches with a pain that interferes with even the simplest of daily chores? If you have parasites feasting upon your body, what meaning can you possibly give to that? If you have survived a horrific car crash, what does it mean that you should be alive, but unable to get up from your bed?

Before we became ill, there were mysteries in our lives that remained shrouded by our limited understanding, experience, and willingness to see. Still, we found meaning, sometimes, in the things we did and were. In the workplace we identified ourselves with a title, a job description, a particular group or company. In our home lives we were "mother," "husband," "sister," "son." Perhaps we identified ourselves by what state we lived in or what region of the country. We could describe ourselves to others by the experiences that we had, "living abroad," "earning a degree," "starting a business." And we even connected our being with how we looked and where we belonged ethnically, socially.

Then, illness struck. Suddenly or over time, a new identity crowded out the ones we had previously enjoyed as our lives bent and snapped from the presence and aftermath of the unwelcome accident, disease, or medical condition. We became a "cancer patient," "lupus sufferer," "paraplegic," "diabetic." To medical professionals we became "cases"; to health organizations, we became statistics. To some outsiders, we became "weak"; to others, we became people to be pitied.

From the onset of a serious illness, we seek to find meaning in our pain, disability, and confusion. Somehow, calling ourselves by our disease or affliction doesn't seem adequate, and labeling ourselves by statistics, or with terms such as "poor thing," is abhorrent to us. We want there to be some noble meaning, some grand explanation to what has befallen us. But as we continue along the way, journeying with our suffering, just when we think we have a handle on what it all means, the answer becomes hidden by something we can't quite see through.

Is searching for meaning, then, the thing to be doing? Or is there something deeper that we need to be focusing on? Could it be that the journey, however mysterious, is the point, and our own willingness to move with the Lord's hand guiding us is the lesson?

After living so long (almost my whole life) with serious illness, I think this is, in fact, the truth of it all. God's judgment *is* "inscrutable," and his way *is* unsearchable.

We might not find *The* meaning in our illness. But we can be sure that, as long as we focus on the Lord in our lives, we will be moving in the right direction.

O Lord, it is human and natural to want to find the
meaning in my illness.
But it is also very easy to get caught up in searching
for it,
when there is so much else to be learned along the way.
Help me to trust you more completely,
to stay on your path,
so that I may live in your light and learn what you
would have me learn,
in all your fullness of time.

ACQUIRING COURAGE

The LORD is my light and my salvation;
whom do I fear?
The LORD is my life's refuge;
of whom am I afraid?
When evildoers come at me
to devour my flesh,
These my enemies and foes
themselves stumble and fall.
Though an army encamp against me,
my heart does not fear;
Though war be waged against me,
even then do I trust.
—*Psalm 27:1–3, New American Bible*

Because of lupus, I hardly know what symptoms might creep up on me from one day to the next. I try to arm myself with precautions, preparation, and perseverance. But sometimes, when I have to have blood drawn, my arm feels fine. Other times, I have a huge bruise and pain that takes weeks to subside. The aftermath of my weekly chemotherapy treatment might leave me incapacitated from nausea and headache, or I might feel only a little twinge. I might wake up in the morning to a raging sore throat, courtesy of shingles that develop overnight, or I might have such swelling in my knees or feet that moving from bed takes major effort.

Living with lupus has been likened to living with a terrorist, and this analogy is true for many other maladies as well. Although some serious illnesses are a bit more predictable, all are subject to those "nighttime raids," those sneak attacks from armies of bacteria, complications, and twists and turns. Many patients feel as though they are on a constant state of alert, armed and ready for a new escalation of "hostilities."

For this reason, the above Scripture verses are so important. Living as we do, at war against disease and affliction, we make as full use of our medical team and own resources as we can. But we also recognize the limitations of modern medicine, the frailty of our own abilities to fight fully against our conditions, and we need to turn somewhere else, too.

What could be better than relying on the Lord? And if we rely on him, why should we fear? He led the Israelites to the Promised Land. He parted the Red Sea. He brought his might down upon scores of enemies. He sent his son, Jesus, and conquered even death itself. Imagine! How much courage that gives us!

Having the Lord by our side as we face the things we hate and fear about our illness is amazingly empowering. Not only do we have all that man can give us, but we have the Lord's support, too. And with him, how can we shrink from "battle"?

Without the Lord, we are missing our ultimate strength, our supreme "commander in chief." But with the Lord, we have might, we have courage.

How can we be afraid?

> *O Lord, even as I suffer from my illness,*
> *I believe in your might.*
> *Even as I am besieged by armies of pain,*

Peace in the Storm

I seek refuge in you.
Help me to feel your presence even more firmly
in my life.
Give me courage to face anything, to endure everything
—with you by my side.

FINDING LAUGHTER

"... God blesses you who weep now, for the time will come when you will laugh with joy."
—*Luke 6:21, New Living Translation*

A good, long laugh is a marvelous thing. It starts out with a chuckle, then builds in intensity and spirit as we break into a great smile. And, if the laughter touches deep within, to the point of tickling the heart, it results in tears springing into the eyes and bringing an overall sense of well-being and fantastic joy. A wonderful laugh is good exercise, too, quickening the pulse, working our abdominal muscles, exercising our lungs and mouths. No wonder there is the saying "Laughter is good medicine!"

Seeing laughter in illness can be difficult. What's so funny about pain? What's so humorous about not being able to walk, to see, to swallow? We equate laughter with good times, and certainly while we are seriously sick, we find it hard to imagine our situation as "good times." I've tried to see the humor in some aspects of my lupus, but sometimes the result is far from funny. My friends and relatives cringe when I speak of my car's handicap placard as "permission to park in the gimp spaces," and I get odd looks when I refer to my wigs as "pelts."

Indeed, some kinds of joking about illnesses and handicaps

34

can be viewed as offensive and tasteless. Children are encouraged not to make fun of those who have disabilities or whose physical conditions are feebler than their own. Comedians who use certain jokes are ostracized. Television and film portrayals of handicapped individuals are closely monitored by advocacy groups and are openly criticized and sometimes boycotted if they are thought to be unflattering. Patients themselves can be viewed askance if they seem to take their illness or physical challenge too lightly, and sometimes even their physicians might not take them seriously if they aren't overwhelmed with the gravity of their situations.

Yes, we "sickies" are encouraged to take illness very seriously, and the society around us does the same. How, then, are we to find the fulfillment promised in the above Scripture and go from weeping to joy? How can we take advantage of that promised "good medicine" and laugh?

Perhaps we cannot see the joy in our suffering, but we can look for it. Indeed, if laughter will not come to us, perhaps we should make an effort to come to the laughter. This can be as easy as watching the antics of a silly cat, dog, or squirrel, or even getting down on the floor (if possible) and playing along.

Our search for laughter might bring us to humorous writing, uplifting music, a fluffy movie. A favorite cartoon, comedian, or sitcom might help us lift ourselves out of our pensive gloom. If we surround ourselves with good friends and family members who uplift us, we are more likely to laugh with them. Children, in all their wide-eyed simplicity, are often very funny. So, too, are older people, whose experience has taught them the value of taking their "lumps" with sugar instead of salt.

If we don't take ourselves so seriously all the time, we might catch glimpses of humorous aspects of our conditions and learn to laugh about them, too. Perhaps you won't be successful in this all the time. But it's worth a try. Remember that laughter *is* good medicine. And it is promised to us, as surely as we will weep, by the Lord whose promises are never broken.

O Lord, help me find laughter, simple and true,
in great places and small, in obvious ways and
unexpected ones,
so that I may be more fully alive
and partake of all of your blessings,
the blessings that you have promised,
that you will never take away.

Surrounded by Angels

Let mutual love continue. Do not neglect hospitality, for through it
some have unknowingly entertained angels.

—*Hebrews 13:1–2, New American Bible*

The postal carrier who delivers your mail. The trash collector who gathers your garbage. The nurse who draws your blood. The friend who brings you supper when you're too sick to cook for yourself. The doctor who squeezes you into his already packed schedule. The stranger who opens a door for you . . .

Each day, in great ways and small, we are surrounded by angels. Not the celestial creatures with halos and wings, but flesh and blood angels who help us and give us encouragement, even if we don't know their names. We might, in fact, never even see them. They might be on the other end of the telephone line when we need help untangling an insurance issue. They could be carefully formulating the batch of medication that we will take to get relief from our pain. They are in the recording studio, composing beautiful music to inspire us. They are seated at their computers, writing words of comfort and joy.

Our angels might be living next door to us or they may be in a distant land. They hold our hands in communal worship, and, sight unseen, pray for us from miles away. Just as we might not know them, they might never know us by name or face, but they include us in their thoughts and prayers—and we are the better for it.

Indeed, we benefit from each gesture of goodwill that is extended to us, no matter where. Angels' actions bring happiness, ease, and peace all over the world, and in so doing, they spread God's love and message of salvation to even the darkest corners of humanity. Conversion happens through them, and renewed hope and purpose. People are strengthened, healed, transformed into angels themselves.

Yes we, too, are part of that wonderful, angelic community.

Take a moment to think of all the angels in your life. Who are they? What do you think of them? How do you treat them?

Perhaps you might be taking some of the angels around you for granted.

What can you do to show your appreciation for them? How can you extend "mutual love" to your angels?

How are you an angel for others?

Recognizing and acknowledging all the angels in your life won't happen overnight. Nor will you be able to reach out to everyone who is in need.

But little by little, day by day, if you realize that you are surrounded by angels, you will see more of them and appreciate them, carrying God's love all around your world.

And in so doing, in entertaining angels, you will become one yourself.

O, Lord, let me not take any act of kindness,
however small,
for granted.
Rather, let me open my eyes and heart to the angels
all around me,
bringing grateful hospitality to everyone,
And spreading your love throughout my life
and your world.

A Peaceful Night

In peace I shall both lie down and sleep,
for you alone, LORD, make me secure.
—*Psalm 4:9, New American Bible*

How is it that the darkness of night amplifies the smallest of noises, twinges, or fears? As you nod off to sleep, the tiniest sense of disquiet can jar you immediately awake and anxious. At such times, questions flood your mind.

Are the doors and windows locked?

Is someone hiding in your closet or under your bed?

Is this shooting pain a signal of something worse to come?

Will you be able to evacuate in time if there is a fire?

In the light of day, some of these concerns seem small. But the night has a way of bringing out the worst in your thoughts, much like waking nightmares that prevent you from finding peace and sleeping at ease. Sometimes, doing something tangible can help you combat your nighttime fears. For instance, you might develop a routine of double-checking the doors and windows, the closets, and under the bed. Or you might leave a night-light on just in case you have to move quickly if there is an emergency. Keeping a telephone and list of doctors' numbers beside the bed is some assurance, as is a supply of medication in case of sudden, debilitating symptoms.

But besides all these tangible things, what else can you do to insure safety as you slip into sleep?

There is something simple, yet very relieving: a heartfelt call upon the Lord.

Bringing the Lord into your nighttime, to stand guard over you and ease your fears, is a powerful way to go from waking to dreaming. For he sees everything, he knows everything, and he wants what is good for each of us. He never sleeps, never even gets drowsy in his watchfulness.

What better guardian could we have than the Almighty?

Who better to oversee our slumber and keep at bay all the "things that go bump in the night"?

Besides his protection, the Lord also brings refreshment. If you trust that he will fend off any worries that prevent you from truly being calm in sleep, you will benefit from deep, restorative rest. Cradled in God's loving arms, you will find healthful, happy slumber.

The next time worries overwhelm you before you sleep, imagine being fully enveloped by the might and protection of the Lord.

Visualize him standing at your door, watching beside your windows, covering you with his strength and love.

Breathe in and out, expelling your worry as you imagine God's peace settling over you.

Relax every tense muscle.

Feel the soft, safe cocoon of your bed receive you and carry you to restful, restorative sleep.

O Lord, my nighttime fears are very real,
but so, too, is your love for me.
Help me take into my heart your desire for my safety,
and bring upon me a nightly peace
that erases all my anxiety and lets me sleep calmly,
to awaken refreshed
and fearful no more.

BEING GOOD TO YOURSELF

So whether you eat or drink, or whatever you do, do everything for
the glory of God.
—*1 Corinthians 10:31, New American Bible*

"No pain, no gain."
Not too long ago, this phrase was a buzzword for effective exercise. The theory was that if you didn't feel aching discomfort while working out, if you didn't push your body to its limits and beyond, you weren't doing yourself any good. This philosophy spilled over into other aspects of life, too. When women became a presence in the workforce, visions of "superwoman" became prevalent, encouraging women to take on grueling multiple roles of professional, wife, mother, volunteer, and homemaker. Even today, stay-at-home moms are often scorned or viewed as having it easy or doing nothing of value with their lives. Men, too, are often depicted by images of "tough-guy" attitudes and activities and can be ridiculed if they give the impression of being "soft."

The "no pain, no gain" philosophy has been adopted by some well-meaning people inside and out of the medical profession, too. Phrases such as "Grin and bear it," "Hang tough," and "Whatever you do, keep a positive attitude" abound. Sick children are sent to day care, adults tank up on cold medications and travel to business meetings. "Everyone's getting that flu bug," is a common refrain—and no wonder! With all the sick people walking around, more people are bound to be stricken!

If society at large seems determined to push through tough physical times, what about those of us who suffer from severe, ongoing illness? How effective *is* the belief in "no pain, no gain" for us? How does it assist us in our day-by-day struggles?

In truth, not at all. In fact, it can hinder well-being. Pushing yourself beyond your already limited capabilities can sometimes cause irreparable harm. Taking on activities, eating nonnourishing foods, or otherwise doing things that work against overall health is anything but what the Lord wants us to do. As he tells us so simply, we should "do everything for the glory of God"—and surely that means being good to ourselves.

If we treat others with heartfelt grace, how can we treat ourselves with anything less?

There is a big difference between indulging in overabundance or shirking responsibility and being good to ourselves; the Lord doesn't mean for us to retreat from what we should or must do. It's the same thing with our daily lives—we need to take care of ourselves, be good to ourselves, before we can be strong enough to be good to others.

Think about the small ways you can be better toward yourself. Can you take an extra fifteen minutes of quiet, just for you? Can you pack a more healthful lunch instead of eating takeout? Can you take a leisurely walk, just "being" in the presence of the Lord? Can you scribble in a journal, your own secret place of personal expression, and let go of the burdens on your heart in calming privacy?

There are other ways of being good to ourselves. They are as personal as we are each individual. But they are vital to each one of us.

Perhaps *our* phrase, instead of being "no pain, no gain," should be "Be good to others . . . be good to yourself."

*O Lord, in the hurry of the day, I often forget
to take care of the wonderful gift of life and self that you
have given me.
Please remind me, in great ways and small, to be good
to myself,
so that I may be ready, willing, and able
to be good to others, too.*

GUILTY FOR BEING SICK

A clean heart create for me, God;
renew in me a steadfast spirit.
—*Psalm 51:12, New American Bible*

You snuggle under the covers of your soft bed, reading by the warm glow of a lamp on the bedside table. You are in severe pain and have just received a not-so-good report from your doctor. But your room is your refuge; it's quiet, peaceful, like being in a protected cocoon.

Suddenly from downstairs, you hear the telephone ring, a door slam, pots and pans clattering to the floor in the kitchen. Your youngest child starts to cry. Your spouse responds with a louder-than-usual voice. Now, your middle child is crying, too. The dog barks. And the telephone continues to ring.

You look up from your book at the stark ceiling, the lamplight glowing less brightly there. Your mind fills with all the things that you *should* be doing downstairs.

The phone is probably the water delivery people. You hope you told your spouse that the order needed to be changed. Dinner should have been ready half an hour ago, because your oldest child—the one running down the stairs—has soccer practice soon, and you were supposed to drive car pool. Will your spouse remember? The dog is due for his shots. . . . Does your spouse remember that, too? And what about that special funny face you make when your youngest starts to cry. . . . Will she resent you for not being there to quiet her tears?

Suddenly, *your* eyes well up with tears and your heart is filled with guilt. If it weren't for your illness, you'd be downstairs in a flash and handle each situation, easing your spouse's burden. But you can't. You're unable to help with these or many other household chores, not to mention not being able to work and so bring even some financial relief to your family.

As you contemplate the many ways you aren't able to help out at home, with friends, or in the community, your guilt becomes horrific.

What have I become? you might ask yourself. *A useless burden to everyone?*

Catholic guilt . . . Jewish guilt . . . Italian guilt . . . Irish guilt . . . It is completely normal to feel guilty about being ill, particularly if you can't carry some of the responsibilities you used to at home or at work. But feeling guilty for too long can bring its own problems, too. Seeing others become overworked because of your inability to work can make you angry with yourself. You might become resentful of what others can do and unintentionally harm your most treasured relationships. Also, you might let your guilt eat away at you and interfere with your healing, which can only compound the problems resulting from chronic illness. Letting guilt distract you from your present job, which is helping yourself heal, is another negative by-product of this.

Yes, it is human to feel guilty, but don't let it go on too long! Remember, our Lord is a forgiving Lord. Just as he forgives us our trespasses, we should strive to replace our guilt of feeling ill with a clean, resilient heart that is ready to do whatever it takes to let him work, to let his forgiveness and mercy show through. Think of each prayer you pray as a way to renew your heart, to cleanse yourself of the guilt of being sick, and to become more steadfast in God's plan for your life. By doing this, you will be able to find ways to be useful—to yourself and to others.

O Lord, wash me clean with your blessed forgiveness
and grace.
Help me to get past my feelings of guilt
so that I may move ahead, along your pathway,
and witness to the many ways in which you work
through me,
because of . . . in spite of my illness.

PRAYER FOR STRENGTH

Awake, awake, put on strength,
O arm of the LORD!
Awake as in the days of old,
in ages long ago!
—*Isaiah 51:9, New American Bible*

Sometimes when you are chronically ill, you don't think you can go another step. All of your inner resources of resilience, fortitude, and strength are depleted. There isn't enough "gas in the tank" to even complain, and you're days, miles away from the proverbial filling station. There is so much to do! But you can't find it in you to move one inch. And as you go farther away from a life of health into a life of illness, you begin to forget what it was like to be well, to be strong and able to take care of your own life.

True, our inner strength can often be horrifically beaten down by physical weakness, pain, and other challenges that we have to meet each day. But we need not despair at times like these. Unique to our lives in faith, we have external strength, which does not diminish like our internal, human strength can. In order to take advantage of it, we have to be aware of it, to "awake" and "put [it] on," as these verses from Isaiah suggest. In our quiet, even at our lowest point, the Lord offers us his mantle of protection, his immense strength. Much like a suit of armor, this gift from the Lord will hold up our fragile selves while we cope with our illness. With it, we *will* have enough energy, hope, and courage to do what we must and fulfill our destiny in him.

Try to picture the "armor of strength" that the Lord gives you each day and night. It is tailored precisely to you, as you are now, and molds to your body even in your suffering. In your mind's eye, see it form a supple yet impenetrable coating of determination. It is not overwhelmingly heavy. It covers you with coolness in heat and warmth in cold. Feel your divine armor imbue your tired muscles with more firmness and your clouded mind with clarity of thought.

As you experience the renewal of direction the Lord also gives, begin to look with fresh eyes toward ways that you can be stronger with the help of other people or products that can make your life more workable. These external things, these extensions of the "armor of strength," are also given to you by the Lord; you need only recognize them and reach out to them to make use of them.

Through small trials and great ones, your armor will sustain you. And as you feel more in control of your life, even with the ups and downs of chronic illness, your protection from the Lord will be absorbed and made part of your heart and soul. You will begin to sense a strengthening *within* much like that outside your body. You will find that you have fewer questions and more tools to solve your problems, and more ease at going about your daily life.

How much more blessed is life with chronic illness if it is lived with the Lord's strength!

Whenever you find yourself crumpling from human weakness, awake! Remember what you have accomplished already. What difficulties you have overcome. Then, call upon the Lord's "armor of strength." Put it on, "as in the days of old," and see just how strong you can become!

Peace in the Storm

*O Lord, in my weakest moments, help me
remember that I am strongest with you.
Let my past accomplishments be an inspiration to me
as I strive to meet the challenges of the day.
And let your armor of strength cover me at all times,
in all ways.*

ANSWERED PRAYERS

"Therefore, I tell you, all that you ask for in prayer, believe that you
will receive it and it shall be yours."
—*Mark 11:24, New American Bible*

The act of praying to the Lord is as fine and old a tradition
as any that we practice today. As regular as the rising and
setting of the sun, we clasp our hands in respectful supplication and lift our voices to God, asking him for things. Release
from pain. A definite diagnosis. More money. Fortitude to resist temptation. Patience with others. A new friend.

Sometimes, though, we lose sight of the purpose of prayer
and behave as if the Lord were an eternal Santa Claus and we,
the children sitting upon his lap, telling him what we want for
Christmas. With wide-eyed expectation, we whisper the exact
size, color, and model of what we want, sometimes even
telling him where he can place the item or attribute when he
delivers it. As we describe what we want, we might cry from
frustration or lean in closer so that "Santa" will take us seriously.

We take our requests seriously. We *want* the things we ask
for. And the longer we pray, the more sure we are that the Lord
will fulfill his promise. After all, isn't this what he tells us he
will do, as evidenced by the above reading from Mark? Some-

times we even set up a time line, thinking that if we pray for so many days (or have a specific deadline to meet), the Lord will comply with our constraints and "deliver" without question.

But prayer is more complicated than a simple session on "Santa's" lap. It is a communication between ourselves and the Lord—something much more complete than what we might take it to be or than we can even understand with our limited human knowledge. For God not only hears the words of our prayers, but he knows us so wholly that he knows what's behind them—that is, what we *truly* need. If, for instance, I pray for a day free from lupus symptoms, he might know that, deep down, I need to be free from *worrying* about the disease, at least for a little while, so he will send a "distraction" that fulfills that need. It doesn't mean that the lupus goes away; the Lord sees me so deeply that he knows more than I do about what I really need.

Only time and staying close to his Word will reveal his ultimate plan.

In all my years of living with illness, I can't say that I have been disappointed by anything the Lord has given me in answer to my prayers. Even in the pain and sorrow, he has revealed wondrous surprises that I would never have received had things always "gone my way." Through it all, I've come to realize that what's more important than praying for specific (and selfish) things is believing that the Lord will give me just what I need when I need it.

I need not desire specifics or be burdened with all the details of them (size, color, etc.) because sometimes I might not have a clue about what's best for me. But I do need to believe, to continue to hold to the fact that he will not leave me wanting, and he will not see me fall.

If we believe in God's desire for our lives and if we truly

pray what is in our hearts, then this belief will always show through. We will see his way for us and reap the full benefits of being his children.

Truly, our fondest wishes and our deepest needs, if we pray for *these* things and *believe* that we will receive them, the Lord promises they shall be ours.

How blessed we are to be his children! How great, how very great, he is!

> *O Lord, you are so great*
> *that you know me better than I know myself.*
> *Even when I pray, my words are empty*
> *because you see through them to my heart,*
> *to my soul.*
> *I know . . . I believe . . .*
> *that you will give me what I ask for in all its fullness:*
> *what is best, what is right, and what is good.*

ALL RIGHT TO CRY

Rejoice with those who rejoice, weep with those who weep.
—Romans 12:15, New American Bible

A year after I was diagnosed with lupus, my brother, my only sibling, died suddenly. His passing was shocking to me, and because it happened out of town and I was struggling with a severe flare, I couldn't even be present in the immediate aftermath, the time when the comfort of family was most needed. Worse, because of another physical problem, Sjogren's Syndrome, my eyes weren't able to produce tears regularly. At a time when my heart was breaking and my soul was in anguish, I couldn't even cry normally. I tried to substitute my lack of tears with crying out in a loud voice, pacing, balling up my fists, even just staring out the window. At times my throat was choked with emotion but my eyes remained dry. At other times the tears did flow, and the feel of them hot and salty on my face was, in an odd way, a great comfort.

I learned a valuable lesson during my time of mourning—a lesson I've carried through to this day: in times of deep pain and suffering, it is more than all right to cry; it is essential. Crying expresses our sorrow in a unique way; it is a symbolic and concrete form of letting our deepest emotions surface and a way to clear our hearts so that we can move ahead. And it is a way for others to know that they can comfort us and be with us even through our pain.

There are many examples of crying in the Bible, two of which strike me most profoundly. The first is in Luke 7:36–50. A "sinful woman" comes to the place where Jesus is dining and, to the horror of those at table, bathes Jesus' feet with her tears, kisses them, and dries them with her hair. Moved with compassion, the Lord forgives all of her sins, pointing out that his host did not give him water to wash his feet nor a kiss of greeting. Truly, in this story we see the wonderful relationship between tears, expressing sorrow and remorse, and the Lord's forgiveness.

The second example that moves me is found in the simple, eloquent phrase in John 11:35. Upon hearing of the death of his friend Lazarus, John writes, "Jesus wept." Even our Lord found expression in weeping! He, in all of his power, cried tears of mourning.

Beyond the obvious in these two examples is something deeper: along with the weeping came reactions of others *and* action on the part of the person who wept. The sinful woman did not just crumble at the Lord's feet and cry, she used her tears to wash his feet. Others around the table criticized Jesus for allowing her to do this, but the Lord forgave her and brought her into a new, cleansed life in him. Likewise, Jesus not only weeps at the news of Lazarus' death, he goes to the tomb and works one of his most amazing miracles: he raises Lazarus from the dead.

Pain, disability, depression, anxiety, loss of a job or a relationship, and other things that are directly related to living with a chronic illness can make us very mournful. So can many of the "natural" things in life: the illness of a loved one, the death of someone close, or other calamity can make us sorrowful, too. For all these, it is all right to cry. In doing so, we express our grief and give ourselves the release we need to move ahead. But perhaps more important, we let others know by our tears that we need their compassion, their understanding and help.

Through the gift of tears we help forge the bonds of love that the Lord made so clear in his divine walk on this earth.

O Lord, I so often feel like crying, yet I wonder
if I should resist in order to be strong.
Please take away my hesitation, Lord, and let me
express myself
with all the gifts you have given—with laughter
and tears.
In expressing my sorrow, let me show others how much
I need them,
and let me be there for them, too, when they are
in need.

STRUGGLING WITH
WEIGHT GAIN

Consequently, from now on we regard no one according to the
flesh; even if we once knew Christ according to the flesh, yet now
we know him so no longer.
— *2 Corinthians 5:16, New American Bible*

One of the most distressing aspects of many serious illnesses is the change your physical self goes through—
especially your weight. Some medications promote weight
gain. Pain can make you unable to exercise enough to burn extra calories. Cravings, too, can contribute to a breakdown in
eating a healthful diet. Misplaced emotions might spur you to
consume large amounts of high-calorie "comfort" foods.

As the pounds pile on, you might become despondent or
depressed over your physical deterioration and, as a result, gain
even more unwanted weight. The longer you go in this cycle,
the more difficult it is to lose weight, and the problem becomes even more difficult to solve.

Denial might set in.

Oh, you understand the difference in your appearance due
to weight gain. You also understand that extra weight puts a
strain on your joints, heart, lungs, and self-image.

But, you might ask, *am I really gaining all that much weight?*

As a child of light and keeper of the precious gift of your body, you know the answer to this question in your heart. Perhaps you need a little prodding to face reality, but you *know* when you're in "weight trouble." (And, if you doubt the reality of what's happening, there are sobering weigh-ins at your doctor's office and written records that reflect the rising numbers.)

The next question, then, is, *"Is there anything I can do about it?"*

Praise our God, there is!

You might not have control over your health condition or the treatments you have to undergo, but you *do* have complete control over what you eat.

Reflect upon this marvelous fact.

Yes, you have control!

It is this connection between control and weight gain that is the most important key to your fight against extra pounds. And it is here that you most need the Lord's help. He *does* know you by name, by physical look. But more important, he knows you *inside*, heart and soul. He knows your strengths and weaknesses. He knows what you need to overcome even your most difficult struggles. And your struggle against weight gain is certainly one of the most difficult.

In your fight to keep the pounds off, reflect on all the external things you use: the diet plans, the counseling, the workouts, the support of others. Add to them regular meditations on the Lord's presence in your life and his love.

God wants you to be strong, he wants you to take the steps that will help you thrive.

He loves you so much that he gave his only Son to be a sacrifice so that you might be saved!

In keeping with the sacrifice Jesus made, pray that you can sacrifice your cravings for unhealthful foods and for help in replacing them with the desire to eat only what is best for you.

Visualize yourself at your most fit and, as you prepare your meals, think of the food that you eat accomplishing this image. Ask the Lord to guide you in this, too, and bring him to your breakfast, lunch, and dinner. Unless your illness demands that you eat snacks, leave aside these foods and "snack" on God's Word and your own quiet time. "Regard no one according to the flesh"; that is, don't compare yourself to the advertised "physical ideals," but dwell on the life and spirit the Lord has given you, and do what is best for *you*.

Making physical changes in your appearance can take a lot of time. But with the Lord's help and his guidance, each forkful and each step, you will be able to shine in his light, and in his image!

Father in heaven, I crave to be a witness for you.
I know that my physical well-being can suffer from weakness.
Help me to keep you in my mind and heart,
and let me take your guidance as I nourish my body
with healthful food and good activity.

You Are an Athlete

I have competed well; I have finished the race; I have kept the faith.
—2 Timothy 4:7, New American Bible

You have never thought of yourself as a particularly committed athlete, but suddenly you've been thrown into running a marathon. At the starting line, you are anxious because you haven't trained enough, nor have you studied the course in advance to know exactly what you're in for. You suspect you will be challenged, physically and mentally, like never before. But now that you are poised to begin, you are determined to finish . . . maybe even run a "personal best."

With a burst of adrenaline, you surge across the starting line and join the throngs of people running on either side of you. You study their running styles, their apparel, even the expressions on their faces, hoping to take from them some tips for making it through. You notice that some people are already far ahead, others are behind. You're about in the middle of the pack, which is fine with you, as new as this experience is.

Not far from the start, you see crowds on the sidelines. They are cheering, waving banners, holding out hands for high fives. You see some familiar faces among them—friends and family members—and this gives you more confidence. You wave back at the cheering throng and give your loved ones a thumbs-up. But your focus on the crowd pulls your eyes from the course. You misstep on a stone and nearly fall. Abruptly, you catch yourself and slow down a little, moving your eyes from the sidelines to the marathoners ahead of you.

You can't finish the race if you don't pay attention to the course!

A mile passes, and then another. You've been doing pretty well, considering your lack of training, but gradually become aware of a strain in your right leg and a dull ache in your lungs. You don't want to stop. So, you adjust your stride a little but push on, truly enjoying the feel of wind against your face and the accomplishment of making the miles slip by.

A few miles more and some of the runners ahead fall back. Some of the runners behind you quit. Seeing this, you gauge your own situation. The strain in your right leg is becoming more pronounced and your lungs are working harder. You want to continue. In fact, you want to overtake some of the runners ahead of you!

But a question forms in the back of your mind: Do you have what it takes to run the full race?

At the start of the marathon, you had more confidence and certainly felt fresher. A lot of people had confidence in you, too. Now you begin to have more doubt than faith. Some of your loved ones have dropped away, and fewer onlookers cheer you on. You have to dig deep to find the personal resources to keep going. In your introspection, a voice inside of you reminds you of what you've already endured.

"Learn from your experience. Learn from others around you who have been running the race, too," the voice says. "See how far you have come already? Now, think of how much farther you can go."

How much farther, indeed! You notice that there are still a lot of people ahead of you and a fair number behind. They, too, appear to be feeling the effects of extreme exertion, but they aren't giving up. Nor will you.

With this inner inspiration, you feel a surge of renewed confidence. Suddenly you feel as if you can not only run the race, you can make it your best ever!

Coping with a chronic illness is like running a marathon. Immediately after your diagnosis, you might feel a surge of energy, determination, and relief that you finally know what is wrong. Although you might be afraid and doubtful of your ability to see your illness through, the support and love given by family and friends encourage you. You begin to follow the course (the tests and treatments prescribed by your doctors) with hope and faith. Then the way becomes more difficult. Your symptoms deter you from fully participating in life's activities. A few of your loved ones become less enthusiastic (or leave you altogether). Your strength fades in the face of treatments, tests, and physical problems. Self-doubt sets in. Your faith flags.

At moments like these, it is very important to reflect upon two things:

How far you've come!

You are not alone!

Indeed, miles are slipping by, and you haven't fallen yet. Your "cheering section," although smaller, is no less vocal. Others are running alongside, ahead of, and behind you and are teaching you and encouraging you with their experience. You are learning how to run with the strains and pains, still eating up ground and getting stronger with each footfall. The way might not be easier, but your ability to cope with it is certainly better. And although you can't see what the course ahead holds for you, you are moving along in the right direction.

The image of athlete is a perfect one for those of us "running the race" of terrible, day-to-day illness. Despite our pains, disappointments, and setbacks, we are being forged in the fire of trial. We are being strengthened. And we are being led by the Lord to the "finish line."

Although we do not know the exact way, if we compete well and keep the faith, we will finish the race—and achieve our personal best!

Heavenly Lord, be my coach and trainer.
Be the wind beneath my wings, the spring in my feet.
Help me stay on the course you have set,
like a strong athlete, a champion,
and let me do my best, always, for you.

Learning to Say "No"

Wisdom reposes in the heart of the discerning
and even among fools she lets herself be known.
—*Proverbs 14:33, New International Version*

"I shouldn't have!"

The stress and effort have caught up with you. You pushed your body too far, taxed your patience, and stretched your health to the breaking point. Instead of feeling fulfilled by what you've just accomplished, you are completely spent. Perhaps you even feel worse than you did before you pushed yourself. Maybe you weren't able to do justice to a particular activity or be as good an employee, friend, parent, or spouse as you thought you could be. Maybe because of your physical frailty, you ended up making a situation worse.

True, you "shouldn't have."

But, you did.

Unfortunately, lost time cannot be recouped. If your health has suffered because you overdid it, you have to take care of the aftermath now. If you made a situation or a relationship worse for your efforts, you have to look for ways to repair the damage.

Above all, now that you see what happens when you do more than you should, you have to learn from your mistake.

You have to learn to say "no."

Not all the time, of course, and not as if you are rejecting opportunities and people as unworthy of your attention. You simply have to conserve your energies for those things that are most important and for those people who mean the most in your life.

Discerning when and how to say "no" is perhaps one of the most difficult things for us to learn when we suffer from a serious illness. There are activities we want to participate in and people with whom we want to spend time. Perhaps we've been the one holding together our family or our workplace. Perhaps we have tremendous responsibility in our volunteer activities or in our places of worship. We know the phrase "To whom much is given, much will be asked," and we have taken it to heart.

But now, we also have to take care of that heart and the rest of our physical selves. Suddenly our priorities must change. But how?

Reaching out to the Lord in prayer is the first step toward truly understanding how we should organize our priorities in light of a diagnosis of serious illness. Asking for the wisdom to know what to do and what not to do, and how to refuse opportunities, is key. Stepping back from outside pressure or our own desires and letting the Lord lead is important, too. There have been many times when I felt weakened by the persuasion of someone who wanted me to do something, but I took a moment to collect myself and allowed God to speak through me to gently but firmly say "no."

Sometimes I don't feel good using this "negative" word. Sometimes I feel like I'm doing the wrong thing by not pushing myself. But I've learned that the benefit of prudent prioritizing is certainly worth it; I have more energy for the things that are truly important and I enjoy them more. Also, I enjoy spending good, quality time with my loved ones. I still make mistakes and am foolish about overextending myself, but I learn from that, too. As long as we seek her, Wisdom doesn't abandon any of us, even if we are foolish.

As we strive to find the wisdom to say "no," we will be doing a great service to ourselves and to others. We will be able to be at our best for the things and people that truly matter.

Yes, you have to learn to say "no."

So that you will be able to say "yes."

O Lord, let me look beyond the word "no"
to understand what it means to my hopes and dreams.
Give me the wisdom to apply this word prudently
and gently
so that I may follow through with those things that
most require my attention and energy.

Waiting for the Treatment/Medication to Work

Cast your cares on the Lord
and he will sustain you;
he will never let the righteous fall.
—*Psalm 55:22, New International Version*

When I was diagnosed with lupus, my symptoms were terrible and getting worse by the day. Joint pain, hands that wouldn't work, excruciating fatigue, pleurisy, frequent infections, an esophagus that wasn't functioning as it should . . . I was overwhelmed.

One of the first medications I was given was Plaquenil, an antimalarial drug. My doctor said it would take "a while" to begin to work. Immediately I started counting the days!

Adjusting to the medication was almost as terrible as my symptoms, and it took three months before I could take it without feeling nauseous. But even after those first months, I didn't seem to feel relief.

"Wait a while longer," was the response. "Sometimes it takes six months, sometimes a year."

Six months! A year! To me, it seemed like an eternity.

Time stretches achingly long when you are waiting for medication or some other treatment to work. Much like the child who "has to go" while on a long car trip, each minute is an hour, and rest stops, like the length of time it takes for medication to "kick in," don't come along soon enough.

No, medications, like those rest stops, come along at their own time.

As I realized that I had no choice, that I truly had to wait, a wonderful thing happened. I put my concern about "how long" in the Lord's hands, asking him for patience and understanding. As I did so, my tension abated and I was able to relax with the knowledge that I *was* making progress toward getting relief, even if I couldn't feel it happening.

With each passing day, there was less time before the medication would start to work. Although I didn't necessarily see results during those early times, I understood that getting better is a process, not something that happens all of a sudden. And I learned to "cast my cares" even more strongly on the Lord.

Finally, after almost a year, I realized how far I had come. In subtle ways the Plaquenil was doing some good. And I was comforted by the Lord's grace, as it flowed into me in exchange for his taking my cares upon his shoulders.

How long time seems when you're in pain and suffering! How long it is, too, for your loved ones, who hope that "any day now" you're going to feel better. Truly, it is like being on a storm-buffeted sea, your boat crashing up and down with the mammoth swells. But when you give your cares over to the Lord, he brings calm.

And when you trust in him, he does bring precious, wonderful relief.

O Lord, help me to understand that you are there
to take my concerns and cares upon your shoulders.
Let me not hesitate to ask you to carry my burden,
and in its place, please bring me calm
to see through the waiting time
to a glorious result.

PRAYER FOR BEING
A GOOD PARENT

"My grace is sufficient for you, for my power is made perfect in weakness." Therefore I will boast all the more gladly about my weaknesses, so that Christ's power may rest on me."

—2 Corinthians 12:9, New International Version

If you are a parent, you know that you have unique challenges in taking care of your children *and* coping with your illness. You can't stop being a parent, but sometimes the weight of your own struggle makes you feel less effective, even less loving, toward your precious children. You might have to miss school events or sports games. You might not have the energy to stay up to tuck your children into bed and kiss them goodnight. You might be so ill that you can't shop for birthday or holiday presents. All of these (and other) "failures" might make you fear that your children will stop loving you, stop looking up to you as "Daddy" or "Mommy," or maybe even dismiss you as their most perfect role model.

But life is not all about being "perfect." Every person in our lives, whether a relative, friend, coworker, or stranger, is a complex mixture of strengths and weaknesses. How dull life would be if everyone were ideal! True, children need people who set examples for them to follow in their own lives. But do those examples need to always be perfect?

Can't children learn from mistakes, unhappy situations, even the serious illness of a parent, too?

Indeed, they can and should.

Your children will be all the stronger for learning understanding of your illness, and benefit from your lesson of persevering in spite of your health challenges and from your reliance on the Lord even in your suffering. They can truly blossom into compassionate individuals under your encouragement to be helpful in your time of need. And they will be able to more fully understand the meaning of "God's love for us."

Of course, how much you ask your children to understand and do will depend upon their ages and maturity. But even the youngest child can gain insight about what it means to be human if gently encouraged and directed.

It is natural to want to be all you can for your children. And you will be, within the constraints of your illness and health needs. Your love for your children will be evident, even if you can't express it in the "normal ways" other healthier parents do. But by looking upon your illness as a God-given teaching and learning tool, you will also be able to bring your children something very valuable that will carry them well in their own lives. You will be imparting the wonderful lesson that love, from a parent and from God, never ends, no matter how difficult the way.

In doing this, your child will become a much more resilient and God-centered person. And you will be a very, very good parent for doing so.

O Lord, please show me the ways that,
in my pain and weakness,
I may be a good parent.
And let your love show through me
to bless my parenting
and my precious children.

KEEPING GOD CENTRAL

Therefore, since we are surrounded by so great a cloud of witnesses, let us rid ourselves of every burden and sin that clings to us
and persevere in running the race that lies before us while keeping
our eyes fixed on Jesus, the leader and perfecter of faith.
—*Hebrews 12:1–2, New American Bible*

To keep themselves from getting dizzy and falling, dancers
and figure skaters "spot" when they do their incredible
twirls and spins. That is, they focus on a point beyond the arc
of their circles and refer to it each time they make a revolution.
In this way, they are breaking the dizzying effect of the spin
and are able to stay on their feet. While they are twirling
around, they don't focus on anything else but the motion and
the "spot," ridding themselves of distractions so that they can
complete moves that awe and inspire the rest of us. And when
they come out of their spins, they are less likely to stumble because they aren't dizzy and can move gracefully along to the
next move, the next spiral.

Living with a serious illness can certainly be a whirlwind
experience. With the extra burden of pain and the challenge of
keeping other activities and responsibilities in life moving
along, it is no wonder that sometimes we fall down, dizzied
and confused about which way to turn next. What a comfort

that we have examples to show us how to prevent ourselves from falling or letting our dizziness overcome us.

At these and other times, we see examples of faithful men and women living graceful lives within the vortex of serious illness. These witnesses know what dancers and figure skaters do: by focusing on the Lord, their "spot," they have the focal point that they need to make it through their dizzying moves to live lives of true inspiration.

No athletic endeavor can be done well without practice. In the same way, our trials serve as practice for our faith and resilience. So, we might not always be in "perfect form," but with our hearts centered on God, we will be more likely to meet the challenges of life with a fair degree of grace and divine form.

In times of confusion, in times when nothing seems to be going well or when you feel all "turned around," imagine yourself as a dancer or a figure skater. Throw off the many distractions that persist in your mind and heart. Keep God central so that you may keep your balance and come out of the vortex with a calm and clear heart.

O Father in heaven, let me keep you foremost
in my life.
Even as the world whirls around me
and I feel completely at sea,
even as I feel pressure and pain,
help me to know that you are the center,
the most important part of it all.
You will not let me fall.
You will not let me stumble.
You will steady my body and soul.
And bring to my life
immense grace.

LOSING YOUR JOB

Job took up his theme anew and said:
Oh that I were as in months past!
As in the days when God watched over me.
While he kept his lamp shining above my head,
and by his light I walked through darkness;
As I was in my flourishing days,
when God sheltered my tent.
—*Job 29:1–4, New American Bible*

One of the greatest joys in life is to be productive. Not only does your work give you an income and self-satisfaction, but it can become a great part of your personal identity. It certainly takes up a significant part of your time!

When you have a serious illness, however, your ability to work can be greatly inhibited. You might even have to quit working altogether, leaving behind your profession, workplace, routine, fellow coworkers, and steady income (with periodic increases in salary) that quantifies what you have done.

More than the tangible things you lose are the "intangibles," the stimulation of work challenges, goal-setting and accomplishments, and personal identity and self-worth. You might find yourself at a loss for what to do between doctor appointments.

You might lament your loss of productivity just like Job did: "Oh that I were as in months past! As in the days when God watched over me."

I certainly lamented when I was diagnosed with lupus. I could not continue working in the job that I had, but I was (and still am) not the kind of person to just sit around. I prayed and prayed for guidance.

Finally, I realized that God was showing me the way the whole time.

Taking care of your health, I discovered, is the priority when you have a serious illness. In many ways, it can become a full-time job, replete with appointments, assignments, and tests. Doctors' follow-ups become "updates," much like employer reviews, and "prognoses" are akin to setting goals and plans for the workplace. Even time spent resting, praying, and "just being" is part of the job description when it comes to taking care of the self, and I discovered that ample doses of each every day are part of the landscape, too.

Beyond the health issues is another vital job: assessing your situation and determining what you are capable of doing and what you want to do with the time and energy that you have now.

Perhaps you really want to change occupations, or perhaps you find you can work only part-time. If you cannot work a "regular" job, maybe you can volunteer (perhaps becoming an advocate for others with your illness). Reaching out to your community is another way to be productive, as is having more time for your own family and friends.

Of course, you will need to take into account your financial situation and other practical matters. But as you grapple with these, lift these up in prayer, too. God knows what he wants you to do, and he will make a way for you to do it.

This process of self-examination, prayer, and researching

can take a long time, but every moment is worth it. Instead of lamenting what you cannot do, you are moving ahead to embracing what you *can* do. How exciting that is!

How like God to make sure that our hands are not idle and our days are not dull!

O Lord, I am the work of your hands.
Please help me find ways to make my own hands
productive.
Let me not be idle but use the gifts you have given me
to make this world a better place,
to bring your Word, comfort, and presence
to all in need—far and wide.

How Much Pain Can I Take?

What strength have I that I should endure,
and what is my limit that I should be patient?
—*Job 6:11, New American Bible*

Everyone has a different tolerance for pain. But at some point during our journey with a serious illness, each of us will wonder the same thing:

How much pain will we be able to endure?

What happens if we can't stand it any longer?

Job wondered this, too.

In his prayers to God, he questioned his human ability to withstand his torments, and as they grew more acute, Job wailed all the louder.

But rather than being disappointing, his anguish is, in a way, inspiring. For as Job cried out, argued, moaned, and lamented his situation, he did not turn his back on the Lord, even though others encouraged (and taunted) him to do so.

Yes, Job remained faithful, trusting in God's presence in his life. And through this trust, Job was brought out of his pain and illness to relief by that very same God.

We, too, are overwhelmed by our pain sometimes. We groan and wail. This is only natural (although sometimes it is very annoying to others). Sometimes we have to consciously give over to the physical reality of what is happening to us.

Voicing our discomfort helps us "let it out" and makes it easier for us to cope.

But our expression does not stop with crying out; there is something deeper in it, something holy and most profoundly sacred.

In our pain, we are sharing something of what Christ suffered when he was nailed to the cross and hung to die. We come closer to the Lord, crossing a bit more of the chasm between our daily drudgery and the Almighty. Our suffering also brings us into communion with the many men and women who gave their lives for their faith or in defense of someone else.

Imagine the implications of this: through our pain and suffering, we are closer to being saints! Through our tears, we understand the suffering of others, even if they live in distant lands. We are able to take on their burden and do something about it, even if it is "only" by praying. We can share our experience with others, reaching out in love and support just as others have done for us. In a very real way, pain brings us more fully into the human family and galvanizes us in a way that easy living would not.

Pain is a natural part of living, like breathing or laughing. There is a certain ebb and flow to it, even if it is chronic. There will be hard times and more restful times, times when we are centered on the pain and times when we have more opportunity to reflect beyond it. In those times, in the oases from the onslaught of pain, we realize that something amazing is happening to us:

In the throes of pain, even with our crying out, the Lord is holding us close to him and bringing us more fully into the presence of the divine.

O Lord, help me to feel your calming hand upon me
when I am in pain.

Peace in the Storm

Let your ever-loving comfort enfold me,
And give me the heart to see
that in my suffering, I am becoming
closer to you . . .
and more divine.

Swamped by "Medical-ese"

Let us then go down and there confuse their language, so that one will not understand what another says.
— *Genesis 11:7, New American Bible*

When reading the information available on illnesses and their treatments, I often think I am reading another language. There are scientific terms for symptoms (hair loss is "alopecia"), medications ("aspirin" is in a drug category called "nonsteroidal anti-inflammatories," or "NSAIDs"), and medical practitioners (doctors who treat nerve problems in the eyes are called "neuro-ophthalmologists") . . . and so on. Sometimes I think everyone should take a class in high school just to be prepared to treat their cold symptoms.

But as mystifying as the language sometimes is, we need to be able to navigate it well enough to understand our conditions, recognize symptoms, and be able to talk intelligently with our doctors. Time to turn to God!

In the Old Testament, after the flood, the people of the earth thought they could build a tower up to the heavens and reach God. In response to their egotism, God "confused" their language, creating many different tongues, making it impossible for the people to understand each other.

But even in his anger, God showed his love and compassion. Rather than eternally dividing the world, he gave the gift of the Holy Spirit. People were able to learn one another's languages and communicate, building bridges of comprehension that have solved many a problem and cemented many a friendship. To this day, many languages are spoken, but there are translators, multilingual people, to bridge the gap between them.

You, too, have the gift of the Holy Spirit. Although you may seem lost in the maze of "medical-ese," you have the ability to understand it and you have the *right* to understand it.

Feel comfortable about asking as many questions as you need to in order to understand what your doctor is telling you.

Ask your pharmacist to explain the implications (and potential side effects) of medication. Read about your condition and search for answers until you find them.

Ask the Holy Spirit to open your mind to this new language. Pray that you will find the right words to convey your questions and concerns accurately—and that your doctor will communicate as clearly back to you.

Word by word, sentence by sentence, you will find a clearer understanding of your whole health picture. And you will find a new way of expressing yourself to your doctor, yourself, and the Lord.

O Lord, help me to not be afraid,
but rather let me eagerly seek knowledge.
Open my mind to the language of medicine.
Give me the courage and patience to pursue
understandable answers to my questions and concerns.
Let me speak clearly and effectively,
and let me comprehend all that is said back to me.

LOSING YOUR ATTRACTIVENESS

About eight days after he said this, he took Peter, John, and James and went up to the mountain to pray. While he was praying his face changed in appearance and his clothing became dazzling white.
—*Luke 9:28–29, New American Bible*

Much to the amazement of his disciples, Jesus was transformed when they "went up to the mountain to pray." Curiously, the Bible doesn't say that Jesus was made "handsome," or "younger," nor does it give the details of the way his face changed (eye color, hair growth or loss, sagging or firmed chin).

The important thing, the miraculous thing, was that he was transformed.

One of my first lupus symptoms was hair loss. Eventually I lost all of my hair and had to wear wigs for almost five years. My hair is still "iffy," sometimes thick and sometimes perilously thin.

I never knew how important hair was until I'd lost it: I sweltered in the summer under my wigs and shivered in the winter. I was initially quite upset that I'd lost my blond hair, and even stomped on the first wig I bought because it was hard to style. Eventually though, I realized that my hair wasn't going to come back anytime soon and I'd just have to adjust.

I made wig-wearing and hat-buying into a game and tried to improve my appearance in other ways to take away from what I'd lost. As I did this, I became *transformed* in a wonderful way—I looked different than I ever had, but I was at peace with the change.

I was determined to be dazzling, and many times succeeded!

When you have a serious illness, you might experience a number of radical changes in your body. Weight gain (or loss). Skin rashes or loss of pigmentation. Muscle atrophy. Loss of a limb. People might seem "turned off" by how you look, and you could become very depressed and withdrawn.

But if you look upon your body changes as a transformation, not as something either bad or good, you will notice a great change in how you view yourself. As you take better care of yourself and pay extra attention to your appearance, you will feel as though you have more control over what is happening to you. You will be more accepting. You will be more confident.

You will be happier.

Your renewed appreciation for your body image will inspire others to be positive about it, too. Their compliments will feed you with an uplifting sense that you are making a good thing out of a difficult thing—overcoming hardship to triumph.

Working with your appearance changes in order to make a "new you" will yield many pleasant surprises. You will discover new colors that make you feel brighter and happier, new textures of cloth that give you a sense of comfort and style. You'll find your deep individualism.

You'll give God more glory the more glowing you become.

Dare yourself to be dazzling! You will be surprised at how wonderful you will feel.

*O Lord, help me to do good things with the
appearance you give me now.
Let me handle this transformation with grace
and humor.
Help me find the joy in the attributes I have,
and let me become dazzling each and every day.*

THE STING OF
UNKIND REMARKS

A mild answer calms wrath,
but a harsh word stirs up anger.
—*Proverbs 15:1, New American Bible*

I was picking up my computer from the service shop and asked the gentleman behind the counter for help carrying it to my car.

"Where are you parked?" he asked.

"Behind the store, in the handicap spot."

Immediately he became angry. "You can't park there."

"I have a placard."

"You shouldn't park there," he snapped. "Only disabled people can use that place."

"I am disabled," I replied, feeling anger bubble up.

"No you're not." He looked me up and down and glared.

"Yes, I am," I said, all my feelings of frustration at having lupus, an oftentimes "invisible" illness, rising into the sharpness of my voice.

"No, you're not. You have no business parking in that space! And you clearly don't need help with that computer." He crossed his arms, apparently deciding that the discussion was over.

I SO want to give him a piece of my mind! I thought. *And I should tell his supervisor. He doesn't deserve his job . . .*

But even as I thought those things, a calmer voice spoke within me:

How should you really *respond?*

People can be wonderful treasures. But people can also be very cruel. Sometimes they might not intend to be that way, but a single word or a phrase from them can really cut us to the core. I have been saddened on a number of occasions because something someone said about my illness or the effects of it on my appearance hurt me. Saddened, yes, and angered. Sometimes I haven't responded to those remarks in a very Christlike manner. I've retorted, expressing my anger in harsh words. When I've done this, the result usually is more anger: the person I'm answering becomes embarrassed about offending someone who's suffering, or else is oblivious to the inappropriateness of their remarks and lashes back out at my anger. More angry words may fly then. More hurt feelings result. It's a terrible, vicious cycle that not only creates pain but increases stress and misunderstanding. It moves us far away from the ideal that the Lord would want us to strive for.

In the situation at the service shop, I really wanted to lash out at the computer technician. Clearly he was way off base to say what he did. But thankfully, I took a breath before I let the exchange of harsh words escalate. I *did* ask to speak to the manager, but instead of berating the employee in front of his boss, I explained, calmly, that it might not appear that I had anything wrong; however, I did.

"Lupus patients often look perfectly healthy," I said, the anger slowly dissipating within me. "But, just like someone who has a heart condition or severe asthma, our disability is not external, but rather internal. I don't need to tell you about the details of my disability, but please understand that my doctor and the people issuing the handicap placard agree that I *need* the ability to park in designated spaces. And I do need help with my computer, too."

The man behind the counter looked at me a moment and then apologized. His supervisor carried the computer for me and he, too, apologized and thanked me for educating them on something they didn't know before.

The whole situation could have been horrible, but instead turned out to be quite blessed. And I learned that I will *always* try to take a breath in the face of unkind remarks and make my answer mild, letting the Lord's compassion and mercy show through.

> *O Lord, be the voice within me that stills my anger*
> *when someone says something to hurt me.*
> *Let me stop my tongue before I utter harsh words,*
> *and instead reflect your love and greatness*
> *in the response I do give.*

WHEN YOU CAN'T GET
OUT OF BED

Happy those concerned for the lowly and poor;
when misfortune strikes, the LORD delivers them.
The LORD keeps and preserves them,
makes them happy in the land,
and does not betray them to their enemies.
The LORD sustains them on their sickbed,
allays the malady when they are ill.
—*Psalm 41:2–4, New American Bible*

Some days, you just can't get out of bed.
Whether it is from muscle weakness, dizziness, or another manifestation of your illness, there are times when you are housebound, bedbound, and unable to go about your daily routine. On those days you might read, watch television, listen to the radio, write in your journal, or just stare at the ceiling. No doubt you count the minutes until you have a visitor or, better still, can get out of bed.

Being confined to your bed can, in many ways, be much like serving a prison sentence. And no doubt like many prisoners, you insist upon your innocence: "I didn't do anything to deserve this!"

Through weeks of recovering from pneumonia and other illnesses in my childhood, I had to learn to not fight the bedbound days too much. I used the time to catch up on school-work, read, write, and dream.

Indeed, having to rest is part of the treatment and healing process of any serious illness, and you certainly benefit more from it if you don't create undue stress by working against it. In a way, being confined to bed is the Lord's way of "keeping and preserving" us; if we tried to drive or do chores or work, we could make our conditions worse and possibly make mistakes or cause accidents, too.

Being bedbound gives us permission to sleep, rest, and, perhaps most important, dream of the time when we will be more productive and more active. Through that dreaming, whether we are able to finally get out of bed or not, we can make plans for our future and determine ways to carry them out. And that positive outlook on the future, that seeing beyond our current trial, is part of the Lord's working in our lives.

"The LORD sustains them on their sickbed,
allays the malady when they are ill."

In our forced confinement, the Lord brings us empathy for others in the same situation. He increases our ability to be "concerned for the lowly and poor." He gives us the means to mend and plan so that we have a purpose, a goal even in our perceived "idleness."

Truly, by giving us our "down" time, the Lord is working within us to preserve us from further harm and help us grow and strengthen from the inside out.

O Father in heaven, you are with me
even when I cannot move from my bed.
Help me to look upon my bedbound state
as an opportunity for coming closer to you
and my fellow sufferers.
Let my dreams take flight, and my health improve,
through blessed rest and cherished quiet.

BEING HUMAN IN A CLINICAL WORLD

Then the eyes of both of them were opened, and they realized they were naked; so they sewed fig leaves together and made loin clothes for themselves.

—*Genesis 3:7, New American Bible*

Can you imagine Adam and Eve going through a complete physical exam and tests in a hospital setting? Those skimpy, unattractive gowns don't leave much to the imagination! Worse, some of the tests are completely dehumanizing, focused only on "getting the right view" of internal organs or "assessing the function" of specific body systems.

In a clinical setting, the person often becomes the "case," and medical professionals might talk about a patient as "the cardiac arrest," "the scleroderma," or "the pancreatic cancer." It is a rare (and wonderful) doctor or nurse who tries to add a bit of humanity to our care; all too often we feel like personality-less, soulless "specimens."

But although we *feel* dehumanized in the medical setting, we are still very human. And we don't leave our modesty, inhibitions, and fears at the door of the X-ray room or the esophageal motility lab.

How do we respond to the clinical way in which we are treated?

How do we find the feeling or humanity in what we have to go through and whom we come into contact with?

There's no easy answer to these questions, only a lot of room for introspection.

Bringing a sense of humor into the hospital or doctor's office helps defuse some of the seriousness and callousness there. Calling attention to anything that makes you uncomfortable and suggesting ways to make the situation better is another possibility. Learning the names of those who are testing or treating you and using them liberally puts a human face on those participating in your care.

Constant prayer can bring a sense of the Almighty into the situation.

Indeed, I make it no secret that I believe strongly in God and Jesus Christ when I am speaking with lab technicians, nurses, doctors, and other medical professionals. I try to bring a sense of humor into all corners of my treatment and remind them if I'm uncomfortable with how I'm being treated. In being so open, I've met many remarkable, believing people. I've also experienced a brightness and a comfort in my care that's refreshing and vital to my own sense of well-being. Where God is present, there is certainly hope and light!

There is nothing that the Lord would like better than to have his creation appreciate and honor the very humanness of their existence. Through our clinical experiences, we can strive to help make this happen.

We can remember not to forget that there is an art, a blessed humanity, at the core of the very real science of medicine.

And we will meet many amazing people, fellow travelers, all along the way.

*Lord, help me to remember that the responsibility to
maintain the respect for my humanity is upon me,*

as much as it is upon the medical professionals
who treat me.
Let me bring your light and love into
all clinical settings,
making my medical care not only scientific,
but wonderfully human.

FILLED WITH GRACE

Finally, brothers, whatever is true, whatever is honorable, whatever is just, whatever is pure, whatever is lovely, whatever is gracious, if there is any excellence and if there is anything worthy of praise, think about these things. Keep on doing what you have learned and received and heard and seen in me. Then the God of peace will be with you.

—*Philippians 4:8–9, New American Bible*

Sometimes it is easy to become very world-weary. When the news is filled with horrible scenes of destruction and death, and our own lives are filled with painful illness, we can feel as if we're being buffeted from all sides by negativity and decay. But just at these moments, we must remember that we are children of light, God's witnesses; we have an obligation to bring joy and comfort to the very world that weighs us down.

How can we prepare ourselves to do this?

The answer is simple, yet difficult to carry out. We must dwell on what Paul says is "honorable," "just," "pure," "lovely," "gracious," "excellent," "worthy of praise." And we must take what we have been thinking on and bring it to the world. Then, Paul says, "the God of peace will be with you."

What is "honorable" in our world today? Where do we find justice or purity? Are there lovely and gracious elements of your life or the world around you?

When did you see or do something that you could say was truly "excellent"? Not "perfect," not "ideal," but "excellent" in the truest sense of the word. Terrific? Noteworthy? Great?

When was the last time that you found something "worthy of praise" and raised your voice to give it its due? When was the last time you complimented your child? Told a neighbor how much you appreciate him or her? Thanked your doctor for the care you receive?

If we surround ourselves with grim pictures of the news and our lives, we will begin to think that that's all there is to the world. But how can this be, if God created it and "saw that it was good"? No, there are marvelous things and people in our world, and it is vital for us to seek them out, to recognize them, and to identify them.

The more you dwell upon things that are good, the more good you will find in your world. You will find that you are what you surround yourself with.

As you fill yourself with all that is honorable, just, pure, lovely, gracious, excellent, and worthy of praise, you will also be filled with a grace beyond all understanding.

And the God of peace will be with you.

> *O gracious Lord, bring me to all that is good*
> *and let me take it into my heart.*
> *Let my actions reflect the marvel and excellence of*
> *your creation,*
> *and through the grace which will envelop me,*
> *let your peace rest upon me now and always.*

SEEING GOD IN THE ORDINARY

Now there was a man in Jerusalem whose name was Simeon. This
man was righteous and devout, awaiting the consolation of Israel,
and the holy Spirit was upon him. It had been revealed to him by the
holy Spirit that he should not see death before he had seen the Messiah of the Lord. He came in the Spirit into the temple; and when the
parents brought in the child Jesus to perform the custom of the law
in regard to him, he took him into his arms and blessed God, saying:

"Now, Master, you may let your servant go
in peace, according to your word,
for my eyes have seen your salvation,
which you prepared in sight of all the peoples.
A light for revelation to the Gentiles
and glory for your people Israel."
—*Luke 2:25–32, New American Bible*

I wasn't feeling well when I went to church a few weeks ago.
I almost didn't go, but something pulled me into my car and
into the restful, dimly lit building. One of the readings was
from Luke, and the preacher reflected on it in his sermon. I
thought he was going to talk about the "glorious day" when Jesus was presented in the temple and Simeon was waiting for
him. Rather, the preacher talked about how Simeon was a holy
man, beloved of god, but not even he knew that one ordinary

day, he would see an ordinary baby . . . and the whole world would be transformed.

I'd never thought about the reading in quite that way. Somehow I'd always thought that Simeon knew a secret, that he was clued in to the Lord's great gift of Jesus Christ. But he didn't seem to know until he saw the baby Jesus that the Messiah was before him. There was no burning bush, no bolt of lightning. Simeon didn't travel through a desert or climb a mountain. He lived his life, kept his faith, and one day he met God face-to-face.

I've never looked at life in the same way since hearing that sermon. God moves mountains, and he moves people. We don't need to go far to experience his power. He is present here, even in the most ordinary of things. What an inspiration that is! Sometimes, living with a serious illness means having to greatly reduce the world around you; but if God can be in the great things *and* in the small, we are in a much better place to recognize him. Cooking, eating, brushing our teeth, talking on the phone with a friend, or standing in line at the store are not just routines, but places and times where we can meet God.

There is so much that is veneer, or surface, in life, but being willing to meet God, to look beyond the surface, can open us up to many amazing surprises.

We are all, in a way, Simeon. We read our Scripture, enjoy our fellowship, spend hours in prayer, and wait and hope in the Lord. Sometimes when we least expect it, the Lord brings us to him and makes our most ordinary lives something quite "extra"-ordinary!

O Lord, I don't need a burning bush or a bolt of lightning
to know that you are near.
Help me to keep my eyes open and my heart respondent
to your presence in the most ordinary things,
that I might grow more abundantly in your grace.

WHEN A CLOSE RELATIONSHIP
FALLS APART

But Ruth replied, "Don't urge me to leave you or to turn back from you! Where you go, I will go. Where you stay I will stay, your people will be my people, and your God my God. Where you die, I will die and there I will be buried. May the Lord deal with me, be it ever so severely, if anything but death separates you and me."

—*Ruth 1:16–17, New International Version*

Ruth's loyalty to her mother-in-law is amazing. In life, sickness, or death, her steadfast spirit was unchanging. How we wish that that loyalty would be with every person that is close to us, no matter how sick we become.

But the sad truth is that our relationships can change drastically when we have a serious illness, and some of them cannot withstand the added stress and challenges that this new condition brings. From our side, too, our priorities are reordered; we have to spend much more time on ourselves, taking care of our health and working with our medical team. Sometimes it might seem as though we see more of our doctors than our loved ones!

Because of the intrusion of serious illness into a relationship, the wedge that comes between a husband and wife, friends, or other loved ones can be terrible, creating a chasm that even the strongest loyalty and love might find impossible to breach. The "better" becomes "worse," the "health" becomes "sickness." Some relationships are not strong enough to adapt. Divorces, breakups, lost friendships, and alienation might add to our pain with losses so deep that they scorch us.

When a loved one steps out of our lives, we mourn, grieving just as if someone dear has died. We feel abandoned and alone. We might be afraid of the future and of developing new relationships lest we be hurt all over again. Naomi, Ruth's mother-in-law, gives us a glimpse of how she felt about her relationship with Ruth, and it shows us how powerful love can be.

Naomi was married and had two sons. But in quick succession her husband and two sons died, leaving Naomi with her two daughters-in-law, Orpah and Ruth. Before Ruth says her timeless words of loyalty, Naomi gives her the option of returning to her family. She expresses how she wants the best for her daughters-in-law and how she wishes them each "a husband and a home in which [they] will find rest" (Ruth 1:9). Orpah does return to her family; however, Ruth decides to stay. Naomi stops pressing the point, "for she saw Ruth was determined to go with her" (Ruth 1:18). And so the two women remained together.

The uniqueness of the loyalty Ruth expresses is not archaic, nor is the love that Naomi showed for her, even telling her she should leave so that she might have a happier life. For good relationships are built upon care, mutual respect, and steadfast loyalty, and there are many such relationships in our world today. Perhaps you will experience loss of one or more close relationships, but you will also be laying the foundation for solid, better ones in the days and weeks ahead. Through your losses you will experience the wonderful loyalty of loved ones and be able to give loyalty and love in return.

Love is vital in every life, and it is especially dear to those of us who have serious illness; we should not, cannot, shy away from it, but rather embrace it in every sense of the word . . . and be ready to do what is good and caring for ourselves and the good of others.

O Lord, when my relationships seem to fall apart,
help me look upon them with fresh, true eyes.
Give me wisdom to let a loved one go,
and courage to embrace those who remain,
with all the loyalty and love that is within me to give.

HIDDEN GIFTS

Since we have gifts that differ according to the grace given to us, let us exercise them.

—*Romans 12:6, New American Bible*

A runner. A jewelry designer. A psychologist. A writer. A mother. A business owner. A patient advocate. A Christian.

These people I know and many others did not start out life doing or being these wonderful things. It wasn't until they were diagnosed with serious illness that they reached deep within themselves and discovered their hidden gifts, abilities that were always there, but were just waiting for an opportunity to be "exercised." Each person struggled with doubt, to be sure; having a serious illness can shake us up so thoroughly that any deviation from our walk toward better health can be frightening. And each also had to face external obstacles to achieving goals. In some cases loved ones objected, fearing that the "patient" was overextending him- or herself. In other cases the change to a new career was so radical that people could not believe that the same person, whom they'd known as, say, an accountant, would have an artistic streak at all, let alone go on to design beautiful jewelry.

All of these changes of career and life did not occur overnight. The runner had to train, carefully and methodically, guided by his medical team. The jewelry designer had to save up for classes and materials and learn by doing . . . and redoing piece after piece. The psychologist had to go back to college, taking courses that she had (gratefully) avoided during her earlier undergraduate years studying fine arts. And the Christian had to overcome her lifelong mistrust of organized religion to find the truth of the Lord's teaching and the wonderful comfort of fellowship with like-minded believers.

Each of these people, and others I've met, agree that finding their "hidden gifts" is one of the best things to happen amid the trial of ongoing illness. They rejoice at their new skills, confidence, and hope, and encourage others to discover *their* hidden gifts, too.

What are your innermost dreams?

Is there something you've always wanted to do, or did as a child, but had to put aside for something more "practical"?

Is there a voice inside of you that's encouraging you to pursue a new avocation, or completely give your life over to the Lord, and you haven't known what to do with it . . . until now?

Your hidden gifts are sometimes obvious, sometimes veiled in doubt or outside pressures.

You have to sit very quietly and pray and meditate on just what it is that the Lord's grace is leading you to do and be.

God doesn't steer you in the wrong direction; over time and with the effort of your willingness to listen, you will know.

And in following his way and making use of the gifts that he gives us, you will be living a life of grace and truth that is amazingly fulfilling.

So, pray.

Reflect.

Reach for a dream.

You'll be surprised at what is within you—just waiting to be let out!

O Lord, help me to recognize the hidden gifts
that, through your grace, I have within me.
Let me make the best use of them,
as you would have me do,
and let me encourage others that this life with illness
has goodness and truth in abundance.

WHERE IS YOUR STAR?

After Jesus was born in Bethlehem in Judea, during the time of King Herod, Magi from the east came to Jerusalem and asked, "Where is the one who has been born king of the Jews? We saw his star in the east and have come to worship him."

—Matthew 2:1–2, New International Version

Have you ever asked for directions and been at a total loss as to understand the answer you got? Without a map, compass, or identifiable landmarks, sometimes even the most determined person can become utterly turned around, and "the short trip" can become "a trek."

Being chronically ill can bring up feelings of being lost, too, especially when you receive all kinds of advice and conflicting opinions (sometimes even differing diagnoses). Quickly, what might have seemed an easy course to follow might turn into a quagmire—and you might be completely frustrated when the sky clouds over and it starts to rain down more symptoms or other problems at the same time.

The Magi had an advantage over other people in their day, especially over King Herod, who wanted to find the baby Jesus. They followed a star, using it as their compass all the way from their distant lands to Bethlehem. Their example of keeping their eyes on that brilliant spot in the heavens while they trod the long road to their destination is an inspiration for you and me:

No matter how confusing the way might be, if we identify

things to guide us onward, "stars" in our life sky, we will be all right.

The brightest star is the Lord, but there are other, lesser ones that can help guide us, too. Keeping our prayer life and meditative life vibrant and active will serve to ground us well. So, too, will having a prayer or an image to call upon when we are particularly stressed that can bring us comfortably to a "quieter" place and thus help us cope better.

There are external stars, too, that we can keep in mind and heart as we travel. A trusted doctor. A support group of people suffering from the same illness. A close group of friends. An advocacy organization. A journal that we keep and refer to to see how far we've come.

Our pets can serve as "stars" that remind us of the simplicity of life and the joy of "just playing." Our children can inspire us with their trust and innocence. Perhaps you know of a place by the ocean or in the woods or meadow that makes you feel more whole; consider that one of your stars and let it lead you to a better spiritual place.

The Lord's presence is in the stars in the heavens and the blades of grass on earth. He is the star of the morning and evening. Our stars lead us away from our distant humanity and direct us to God's glory, power, and comfort. Knowing where they are and what they mean to us will give us hope and brightly, wonderfully, light our way.

O Lord, let me recognize the stars in my life
and help me to follow them all the way to you.
When I feel most lost,
let me remember them,
and when I am most confused and despairing,
let your stars be beacons that bring me fully,
firmly,
to you.

WORRY THAT YOUR CONDITION
COULD GET WORSE

"So don't worry about tomorrow, for tomorrow will bring its own
worries. Today's trouble is enough for today."
    —*Matthew 6:34, New Living Translation*

When you were first diagnosed with your illness, no
doubt you heard of similar cases and some "horror stories" of people who did not do very well. I still hear tales of lupus patients who died quickly and unnecessarily, or of "lupies"
who couldn't avoid losing all their kidney function. In fact,
when I was first diagnosed, my doctor suggested I *not* go to
support groups because the people there might be so far ad-
vanced in their disease that it would depress me.

What, me, worry?

All right, I confess that I can be a worrier. Oh, I know it's
not productive or good for me. Worry, I've found, eats up precious energy and steals my focus from what I should be pay-
ing attention to. It also weighs down my spirit and causes a
tension inside that interferes with my ability to clearly hear the
Lord's calling.

Worrying does teach valuable lessons. . . . I only wish I'd
learn the first time around! Sometimes, for example, I've worried about things that turned out to be not worrisome at all.

I've feared side effects from new medications and had none. I've thought blood tests would come back showing a new problem, and they did not. By carefully investigating more than one pharmacy, I found one that would serve my needs— so I didn't need to worry that I'd have to struggle with subpar service. I try to remember this lesson each time I start to worry about a new problem. And it works . . . sometimes.

The physicality of worrying is another thing. For example, I do my best worrying lying in bed. But wouldn't it be so much better to spend that time sleeping or at least relaxing? Taking a walk while worrying spoils the beautiful day and can even trip me up if I'm not watching where I step. Worrying tightens my throat and neck muscles. It exhausts me. Sometimes it even makes me itch! With lupus I have enough physical symptoms. . . . I don't want to add to them . . . or *worry* that I'll add to them. So, I try not to . . . and sometimes I succeed.

The more people tell me not to worry, I do. I can't help it. It's something like an "opposite trigger phrase." My doctor might tell me, "Don't worry about losing more hair." I'll count the strands in my brush. I *want* to believe people when they tell me there's nothing to worry about, and I do . . . sometimes . . .

I strive for the ideal in the reading from Matthew, and I know others do, too. But to some of us, worrying comes naturally and is a hard habit to break. I work extra hard to lift up this part of my life in prayer . . . each and every day.

The course of lupus is unpredictable. Some people do quite well, while others have worsening disease despite all efforts to prevent it. Naturally, I have wondered what my case will be in the years to come, and within that wondering is sometimes a healthy dose of fear. I do my best to take care of my medical conditions and live a good life. Right now I can't imagine having a worse case of lupus, but what if someday I do?!

So, I go back to the reading from Matthew. I do take its meaning to heart. I know that ridding myself of worry is a work in progress—and I'm grateful that the Lord loves me and has a lot of patience!

O Lord, thank you for your blessings in my life.
Help me to focus on them and not worry about
tomorrow.
Let me do my best to meet today's challenges
and learn from my mistakes
so that I will transform my spirit
and appreciate your life and creation all the more.

ADVOCATING FOR YOURSELF

What then shall we say to this? If God is for us, who can be against us?

—*Romans 8:31, New American Bible*

When you feel awful, one of the most difficult things to do is to have to fight for yourself. Calling the insurance company, for instance, can be a heavy burden, especially if you get someone on the phone whose purpose is *not* to help you. Dragging yourself to the emergency room in the middle of the night and navigating the bureaucracy to convince the hospital staff to take your complaints seriously and promptly can call for a herculean effort that you might not feel is possible.

Yet, the one closest to your medical condition, and the person who has the most invested in your health, is you. Your loved ones and doctor can provide some support and assistance to you, but sometimes you must strive to overcome your fatigue and pain to advocate for yourself.

Thankfully, we have the Lord in our corner. Many times, I've experienced his power when I've felt too weak to stand up for myself. Even before I was diagnosed with lupus, he guided me through the mystery of my symptoms and unconcerned doctors to give me the strength and words to demand diagnostic tests to determine what really *was* wrong. I couldn't have done that for myself; I was sinking fast because of my illness. I needed his involvement, his soldiering for me . . . and received it in abundance!

Praying for the Lord's protection has served me remarkably well when I've been faced with unsatisfactory healthcare. Not only does he know what I need, he follows through, moving even the most stoic of hearts.

Once I had to undergo an arthrogram procedure, and it wasn't conducted well at all. Afterward, the medical "team" left me on the table instead of helping me walk to the waiting room. I lay in pain and frustration, praying for help. My prayer was answered in no time when a nurse happened upon me and steadied my step back to meet the friend who was waiting for me. If she hadn't come along, I'd have been there for a very long while!

With God for us, we can relax when it comes to talking with people who have to do something for us.

Who can be more forceful than the Lord?

All the shouting or threatening we could do are nothing compared with the power of our God! We simply have to present our needs, politely insist upon them, and persist until we achieve the desired result.

The Lord is all the "muscle" we need.

God's might can fill us with energy we didn't know we had, and hope of the right kind of care at just the right time. His presence in our lives gives us the ability to do what we must every day: advocate for ourselves. The next time you are world-weary and wonder where you will find the strength to carry on, call upon the Lord. A better ally cannot be found!

O Lord, be with me as I work through
all my healthcare issues.
Through your power and wisdom,
give me the strength to advocate for myself,
even in the most difficult of situations.

FINDING A WAY TO DANCE

You have turned my mourning into joyful dancing.
You have taken away my clothes of mourning and clothed me with joy,
that I might sing praises to you and not be silent.
O, Lord my God, I will give you thanks forever!
—*Psalm 30:11–12, New Living Translation*

The Arthritis Foundation has a wonderful exercise program called PACE, which stands for "People with Arthritis Can Exercise." I've attended a few workshops where PACE was taught and each time was amazed at the way exercise can be adapted to people of various physical capabilities. People who cannot get out of a chair can benefit from PACE in a very aerobic way. People who have trouble moving their hands or arms can usually find *something* to exercise and get terrific results.

I, who used to use any excuse to get out of high school gym class, actually enjoy it!

Taking my newfound enthusiasm for exercise, I've also looked for ways to bring a physical expression to my feelings about the world around me and God's love. Sometimes I find myself lifting my arms, stretching, and actually dancing for the joy that God brings into my life. No one sees me . . . except God. I don't necessarily need music or the "proper" dance attire; I just need to extend the love for God that is in my heart and *move*! In fact, this uplifting movement is an extension of prayer, a way of giving praise from me to my Lord.

I always feel better after my little "dance" sessions. My body appreciates the exercise and my spirit is rejuvenated. Also, I experience God's return of my love in the sense of well-being and pleasure that my dancing brings. After all, what parent doesn't enjoy their child's fledgling attempts at dancing, no matter how awkward?

There are many times when I am not able to walk without pain, or am confined to my bed. Even then, I can't stop dancing. I might only be able to gently rotate my feet or curl and uncurl my fingers, but in each "step," I'm still expressing my joy at being alive and what a miracle God's creation is.

How can we be silent, with the Lord in our lives?

How can we stay still, with the Lord's spirit moving within us?

No matter our physical problems, no matter the time of day or the mood we're in, God's awesome love and power invites us to speak, pray, sing . . . *dance*.

And before our audience of The One, we will always receive a thundering ovation!

Father in heaven, thank you
for all that you have given me,
especially for turning my mourning into dancing.
I want you to know that,
even if I am not graceful,
I am profoundly, joyfully grateful!

ON THE EVE OF SURGERY

Even when I walk through a dark valley,
I fear no harm for you are at my side;
your rod and staff give me courage.
—*Psalm 23:4, New American Bible*

As you face surgery, there is no better time to call upon the Lord's protection. In your unconscious state, you will have no control over what goes on. Your medical team will be working. Your friends and family will be praying. But you will be far and away, beyond any active involvement in what's happening to you.

Before you "go under," it is natural to be fearful. You might wonder if you'll come out of the surgery all right, or if there will be some mix-up or mistake during it. You might also worry about what the surgery will reveal about your overall physical state and whether there will be other illnesses or if you will have trouble recuperating. If you don't have adequate insurance, you could also be tense about the financial ramifications of surgery and a hospital stay. Or you might be troubled about who will take care of your family or other responsibilities while you are unable to.

All of these fears and worries contribute to your heightened sense of mortality and helplessness. They bring on stress. They distract you from your spiritual strength.

At times like these, you most need to stay close to your prayer life, your faith, and God.

Undergoing surgery is much like walking through a "dark valley." This is why I think this reading from Psalms is particularly powerful for when you face surgical procedures. Repeating it, reflecting on the spirit and help it conveys, can gently turn your heart from troubles to a galvanized courage that leads to peace and readiness.

No matter what occurs during your operation, you *know* that you will not be harmed.

You *know* that God is with you.

You *know* that he gives you his rod and staff, which are the means to finding your way through the darkness back into his light.

When we have surgery, we put our trust into the hands of our doctors. In the deepest sense, we have no control over what will happen. We believe that our medical team's experience and knowledge have prepared them for operating on us, and we have faith that the outcome will be as intended.

But more important for our own spiritual nurturing, we have faith in the Lord that we will get through the surgery with our souls, our hearts, focused on him and our courage strengthened by the ordeal, no matter what the outcome is.

We must trust our God to do what is best for us at all times.

Truly, when we walk through these "dark valleys," we *can* fear no harm.

With the Lord by our side, and with his guidance and protection, we will stay close to him and see our way through . . . to remarkable, redeeming light.

Maureen Pratt

O Lord, as I face surgery,
you know what my fears and worries are.
Please guide my heart and soul to trust in you,
to know that you are at my side and pouring your
protection upon me,
even through the darkest valley.

LIVING A DIVINE LIFE

You who dwell in the shelter of the Most High,
who abide in the shadow of the Almighty,
say to the LORD, "My refuge and fortress,
my God in whom I trust."
—*Psalm 91:1–2, New American Bible*

I s nothing sacred in this world of ours today? Have manners fallen by the wayside? Are conversations so open that nothing is too taboo to talk about? Do we *really* need to know everything about everyone? Do we *have* to swap health horror stories as though we're talking about the weather or our summer gardens?

Where is the divinity in the world around us?

Where is the divine life for us?

It might be hard to find the divine in the world, but it is possible to build it in our own lives.

Possible, yes, and very important.

A serious illness leaves nothing to our imaginations in regard to the function of our body's organ systems, the way medications and treatments work, and the effects of our illness on our lives. I've lost count of the times that I've been privy to conversations among lupus patients, or others suffering from chronic illness, and the talk has escalated into a "can you top this" of how painful, gruesome, or disgusting an individual's health can be. In a real way, the more you live with an illness, the more immune you become to how ugly such conversation can be to outsiders. I think we've all had occasion to stop ourselves just in time before mentioning a health issue at the dinner table!

In the midst of this morass of harsh realities, clinging to something of the divine is vital to giving our lives beauty and spiritual sustenance. Truly, we must strive to "dwell in the shelter of the Most High" while existing on a human level here on earth. To not do this means that we have given in to the world, to the concrete things around us, and have closed off an essential part of our very being, our soul.

And in doing this, we die a slow spiritual death.

Each of us has individual ways of more fully living a divine life. For some, simplifying the clutter around the house or taking more time for quiet prayer can help. For others, creating uplifting works of art is important. Some people find that giving to others helps them put their own illness into perspective, for in doing so, they are bringing a bit of the Lord along, too. Other people feel more connected with God, and thus more holy, by working the soil and growing beautiful flowers.

If you think of yourself as always living in the Lord's house, of abiding in the shadow of the Almighty, you will find a way to live a more divine life. It helps me to ask myself, "What do I want to say and do in the Lord's house?" This immediately brings my actions and words into the context of God, into the presence of the divine. Many times I have altered my intended actions or words because I knew they would not fit in this more blessed place.

As you think of what you do and say, think of how you are living "in the shelter of the Most High." The Lord is your refuge and fortress.

How fitting that we should strive to live as divinely as he would want us to!

O Lord, it is easy to become "of this world."
Help me recognize where I truly dwell, in your shelter,
and where I truly abide, in your shadow.
And let my actions and words reflect all that it means
to truly live a divine life.

LESSON FROM JOB

If only I knew where to find God, I would go to his throne and talk
with him there. I would lay out my case and present my arguments.
Then I would listen to his reply and understand what he says to me.
—*Job 23:3–5, New Living Translation*

Doesn't Job sound reasonable in the way he wants to go to
the Lord and resolve his problems? Why, it almost seems
as though Job thinks of his relationship with the Lord as a
business proposition or professional arrangement; his manner
of seeking to understand the Lord's intent is certainly very
methodical.

But, as we know, the Lord transcends what is merely ra-
tional. Faith, in its very essence, is the "belief in things not
seen," and our walk with the Lord is not "logical," at least not
to us. Moreover, we know that we do not have to seek the Lord
in some far-off place; rather, he is all around us, even within
ourselves and others. We need only still our hearts and listen
to hear his voice.

How many times have you thought over how you would
tell someone you didn't like what they were doing? Over and
over, you'd turn the problem upside down and right-side back
again, considering all the angles of your argument and preparing for all kinds of responses from the other person. But when
you actually talked with the person, did things go exactly as

you'd planned, or was there an element of surprise in their re-action to you and their answer? Probably, there was something you could not have predicted about what they said to you.

If people aren't completely predictable, then how can we expect the Lord to be so?

Aren't we better off trusting him and spending time in prayer so that we can let him come to us and reveal his plan for us, in his own time?

Job's desire to be active in seeking out the Lord and putting forth his concerns is admirable. We can't just sit idly, without focus, and expect the Lord to hand us his wisdom without inviting it. But Job's expectation of what should happen next is something else entirely. He thought that if he approached the Lord and presented his case, there would be a back-and-forth kind of exchange that would reveal the Lord's meaning. This is a very human way to think of God, but it lacks one crucial ingredient: the almighty essence of how the Lord works to lift us up, to encourage us to be "like him."

In my classes in linguistics (the study of language), I learned that words are symbols for things, feelings, concepts. By putting something into words, you are limiting yourself, in a way, because you are making abstract things concrete. Think of the phrase "I can't put into words how I feel," and you'll know more clearly how imperfect Job's attempt at under-standing God really is. He wants to put it all into words, finite symbols, whereas the Lord is blessedly infinite.

As you think about the way you go about understanding how God responds to your prayers, encourage yourself to go "outside the box" of simple human conversation. Seek the Lord within yourself as well as in the world and people around you. Don't worry about finding *the* place of God; he is close at hand. Strive to hear the Lord in nonlinear ways; that is, instead of expecting an exchange of "I say," then "God says," *listen* without speaking, *feel* God's words without spelling them out

concretely. Above all, *know* that God is beyond our full understanding, but *trust*, too, that he loves us more dearly than we
could ever put into words.

Father in heaven, I strive to understand you
in a way that is imperfect, at best.
Still my futile efforts and instead open my heart
and ears
that I may hear you with a clear soul
and have faith in you beyond my limited knowledge.

PRAYER FOR CHILDREN WHO ARE ILL

Jesus, however, called the children to himself and said, "Let the children come to me and do not prevent them; for the kingdom of God belongs to such as these."
—*Luke 18:16, New American Bible*

Before I was eighteen years old, I'd had pneumonia thirteen times. I'd been hospitalized several times, which was a terrifying trauma for me, and endured weeks away from friends and school. Throughout my illnesses, I relied on the care of my wonderful mother and many doctors and nurses. And I turned to prayer. The comfort from that time with the Lord sustained me even when nightmares crowded my restless sleep.

Today I feel a special burden for children who suffer from illness. How well I know what they have to cope with! They must learn about their bodies and their mortality at a much earlier age than their peers. Illness can prevent them from keeping up in school and stop them from participating in sports and other activities, social and school-related. They miss the very things that make wonderful memories later.

When a child is ill, the world can often feel as though it is suffocating the natural joy, hope, and innocence that should be hallmarks of childhood. Pain can cloud dreams. The very act of having to labor at breathing, not knowing if there will be another puff of sustaining air to fill the lungs, can be horrifying. Loss of limbs, sight, hearing, or other vital functions can curtail discovery of all aspects of our very wonderful world.

For adults, time passes with increased speed. But for children, well, have you ever heard a child lament that Christmas or a birthday is "too far away" when it's only the next month? Time for the child who is seriously ill moves at a snail's pace, if at all. Health and normal activity seem eons away, if attainable at all.

The psychological ramifications of being ill as a child are difficult to quantify, but they exist. Children who are sick might be viewed by their peers as being weak, different, or useless. Getting behind in class work can create a sense of futility; chronically ill children might think that no matter how hard they try, catching up and doing better academically will never happen. They might seem odd to adults, too; the seriousness with which they have to approach their lives is reflected in all that they do and say and gives them a sense of being old beyond their years.

Some illnesses can affect a child's development and physical capabilities. This, too, can reflect upon that child's self-esteem as well as future plans and dreams. Travel, even school field trips, might appear to be too risky to participate in. The child might become overly protective of his or her health and miss opportunities to grow and learn.

The world today is a very different place from when I was growing up. I can only imagine that, with all the terrors in our society, even healthy children have an edge of wariness and fear that tinges their lives. The child who suffers from illness certainly must feel this tension, too, and, added to the already heavy burden of sickness, must feel especially anxious.

To be sure, there are wonderful things I learned from being ill. I am closer to the Lord, for all the time I spent in prayer as a child. I am more sophisticated about my approach to healthcare and my own capabilities. And I think that having been so very ill so very young has put me in a unique position to pray for children who are suffering now.

You, too, through your experience of illness, share something unique with children who have serious illnesses. And your prayers will help give them hope and bring them closer to the Lord, even if they feel that time is passing by too, too slowly.

O Lord, let your comfort and strength
be upon all children who suffer from illness.
Please bless them with your light,
and let them know that they are loved by people
near to them
and united with them in like-suffering and like-faith.

MOVING SLOWLY IN A
FAST-PACED WORLD

LORD, my heart is not proud;
nor are my eyes haughty.
I do not busy myself with great matters,
with things too sublime for me.
Rather, I have stilled my soul,
hushed it like a weaned child.
Like a weaned child on its mother's lap,
so is my soul within me.
—*Psalm 131:1–2, New American Bible*

Each time I am made to move slowly because of my illness, I am reminded of the Aesop fable "The Tortoise and the Hare" with its moral: "Slow and steady wins the race." To recap the tale, the hare and the tortoise decided to have a race. The hare, of course, took off quickly, leaving the tortoise behind in the dust. Step by step, though, the tortoise plodded on. Somewhere during the race, the hare decided to rest. He fell asleep. The tortoise kept going, step by laborious step. And he passed by the hare, finally winning the race!

This story is quite inspirational for me, especially when I'm made painfully slow by illness and can't hope to keep up with others who are healthier, darting from here to there, working and living up a storm. I think I am the tortoise, steadily moving along, not overtiring myself and not losing focus on the path on which I'm treading. When I do speed up or take on too much, I quickly feel the effects in my health and spiritual well-being . . . and I remind myself of the tortoise and try to pull back.

Of course, there are other emotions at play when you see the world moving quickly all around you, but you can't keep up with it. Sometimes you think you're missing out on exciting, important events and activities. You might resent others who are more able than you. You might force yourself to try to keep up and do yourself harm in the process.

Being slow in a fast world can be limiting, but it can also open up other avenues of experience and life that the faster mover misses. Thinking of the hare, again, consider his frantic pace and loss of momentum; all he could do was run and sleep, whereas the tortoise was able to experience the path in all its fullness, from start to finish.

And then, there is this thing about winning. . . .

For us, the prize at the end of the race is not exactly the point; as Christians, we already have our prize in salvation through our Lord Jesus Christ. But there is a kind of triumph at being able to keep on the path the Lord gives us, minding our steps and the surrounding countryside and coming home at the end. And there is certainly a reward more precious than any gold medal:

By moving slowly, giving our souls time to be quiet, we can find our way more assuredly to the peace and comfort of our Lord.

It is hard to be still in the midst of a worried world. All sorts of traffic from cars, people, events, responsibilities conspire against being "hushed." When you are ill, it is even more of a challenge to find a quiet place; a stretch of uninterrupted, pain-free time; and the attention to keep focused on the peace within. But because of the benefit of this most precious gift, it is something to strive for and to encourage others to do.

Indeed, I suppose one of the biggest differences between our walk through life and that of the tortoise is that we shouldn't pass up the hare, letting him sleep; we should witness to him and invite him to join us in our travels with the Lord. And, of course, show by our example of calm that even with the greatest challenges, it is possible to be slow and steady . . . and "win" the race!

Lord, I sometimes worry that the world is
passing me by,
that I am missing out on many things because
of my illness.
Help me to see the good in the pace that you give me,
and let me be peaceful, in you,
throughout the "race" of life.

MANAGING EXPECTATIONS

> Some men came carrying a paralyzed man on a sleeping mat. They
> tried to push through the crowd to Jesus, but they couldn't reach
> him. So they went up to the roof, took off some tiles, and lowered
> the sick man down into the crowd, still on his mat, right in front of
> Jesus. Seeing their faith, Jesus said to the man, "Son, your sins are
> forgiven."
>
> —*Luke 5:18–20, New Living Translation*

Now, here is one determined patient! He's paralyzed, he's
overwhelmed by the crowd surrounding Jesus, and he
goes to the *roof*?! What's more, he trusts his friends to carry
him there and lower him down to Jesus. *That* is faith! Some
people would view the first obstacle, the thick crowd, as a kind
of "sign" that they weren't supposed to see Jesus anyway. Actually, some people wouldn't even make the effort to *go*! But
this man truly takes chance after chance.

And the first thing Jesus says to him is not, "Son, you are
cured." No, Jesus says, "Son, your sins are forgiven."

Do you think the paralyzed man is overwhelmed with
thanks? After all he's gone through to get to Jesus, he's probably stunned that the Lord doesn't heal him, at least not right
away. Finally, of course, he *is* cured and takes his mat and walks
home.

But Jesus' first words to him couldn't have been reassuring.

After all, the man wanted to be *cured*!

We all have expectations when we go to our doctors. We prepare lists of medications, questions, and symptoms. We endure long moments (or hours) in the waiting room. We suffer the indignity of taking off our clothes and putting on those oh-so-charming gowns. We're poked and prodded and stabbed. And *we* pay for it!

After all this effort, we expect results. But sometimes we don't get exactly what we expected. Sometimes our doctors don't seem to pay attention to us, or take call after call during our appointment time. Other times our questions go unanswered or the doctor "doesn't know" what to say or do.

We might get all geared up for receiving a firm diagnosis of what's been ailing us, only to be told there are more tests to run or specialists to consult. Disease progression or the length of time left to living could continue to be mysteries to us and our physicians even after an exhaustive examination.

We're not the only ones affected by unmet expectations; our loved ones want to know as much as we do "What's wrong?" "What can you do for it?" "How long will you suffer?" Just like the friends of the paralyzed man, our family and friends are with us through our appointments, in spirit if not in body. And they want to know, too.

Looking at this instance from Luke again, however, the paralyzed man was actually more blessed than he probably recognized he was at the time. Jesus, our Lord, could have cured him right away, just as he had other people. But by first forgiving the man's sins, Jesus was making a very important point:

The health of the soul is first. That of the body will follow.

If we consider this as we prepare for our doctor visits, the process becomes less burdensome. We still write down our lists, we still have to wait and wear those gowns. But our expectation is less urgent and more accepting, and also more productive. If we have to have more tests run before we get answers, we will. If we have to see a specialist, we will do that, too. If our doctor does not pay attention to us, we'll mention this and either work with the situation so that it gets better or seek another physician who is better focused.

Our expectations, in short, should not stop with the physicality of our doctor visit, but rather extend to the condition of our souls and emotions.

Without a clean soul, the paralyzed man would continue to be spiritually paralyzed. No matter how much he could walk, he wouldn't get very far. But with the Lord's forgiveness, the man is completely ready to live his life, to "go home" and be a witness.

All his preparation was not in vain. It was but the beginning of a new and exciting process.

And so, too, it is for us.

Lord, as I prepare the physical things that go into
an appointment with my doctor,
please let me be in the right frame of mind
to do what is best for my health, body and soul.
Be with me.
And let me not be frustrated, but heartened, by the
ongoing process
that is health-seeking and forgiving.

LETTING GO OF DENIAL

Then Job began to tear his cloak and cut off his hair. He cast himself on the ground and said,

> "Naked I came forth from my mother's womb
> and naked shall I go back again.
> The LORD gave and the LORD has taken away;
> blessed be the name of the LORD!"
> —*Job 1:20–21, New American Bible*

Before being diagnosed with a serious illness, people sometimes experience a decline in health. It might start out as a general malaise, a kind of "blahs" that isn't specific to certain symptoms. But as the illness grabs hold, more things seem to go wrong. Finally, we seek a doctor's opinion and start on the road to a diagnosis.

Along that path, as we undergo tests and examinations, there is a part of us that hopes, even doubts, that there is something terribly wrong. Denial is quite common among newly diagnosed lupus patients, as it is, I'm sure, among others who are just beginning to come to terms with having a chronic, serious illness. It is much like the feeling you might have if you stumble on a high ridge and lose your footing. You scramble to stay on top, kicking at the soft earth and gripping it with your hands, but still you slide over the edge. As you do, you grab hold of a tree and pray that it holds—that you won't fall into the unknown territory below. But you know it is just a matter of time before you fall . . .

It is just a matter of time until you have to let go.

Some degree of denial is very important at the beginning of a serious illness. It allows you to digest what's happening to you in smaller bits and helps prevent you from being shocked into inertia at the reality of your diagnosis. It also enables you to learn what you need to know about your condition and how it will affect your life in a way that helps you make gradual changes.

But clinging to denial, just like clinging to the tree, is finite in duration. Eventually you will have to accept what is happening to you and move ahead with it.

Eventually you will have to let go.

Job's response to the effects of his misfortune is remarkable; he acknowledges God's greatness and power, and he fully comprehends that it is the Lord's will to "give and take away." Then, and the most remarkable thing, Job *praises God* in spite of his suffering!

On the face of it, this positive affirmation of the greatness of the Lord seems out of place. Shouldn't Job bemoan his plight? Shouldn't Job question why a loving God would allow such terrible things to befall him? Or, shouldn't Job have argued about what was happening to him, even arguing that he didn't deserve it?

If you look beyond the obvious, you will see that instead of being out of place, Job's response was *exactly* right. For he knew that the Lord's power was greater than anything he could argue or complain about. He knew that he came "naked" into the world, and that he owed all of his life, even what was taken away, to the Lord.

In these verses, Job truly lets go of his human misgivings and puts himself squarely in God's hands. In doing so, in praising the Lord, he injects an energy and a hope into his situation that echoes through the ages as an example of how we, too, can rest in the Lord's decisions for our lives and have the courage to strive beyond our denial to productive action. Even if the illness and pain are difficult for us to accept, they *are*. And the Lord is still with us as we let go of our denial and embrace the rest of our journey.

It is very true: we didn't come into the world with much. Only everything. Oh, we didn't have clothes and a house, a job, and all kinds of things when we were born. But we did have, and still do have, a place at the table of the Lord, a soul and a name that are known completely by God. We might have to give up a lot, to let go of our life before illness. But we will never have to let go of the Lord.

As I go from health to illness, Lord,
I am fearful that I will not be able to withstand
the journey.
Help me to trust in you completely,
and be my support and strength as I let go
of all denial and accept my situation
so that I can do something positive about it.

FEAR OF AGING

Do not cast me aside in my old age;
as my strength fails, do not forsake me.
Restore my honor;
turn and comfort me.
That I may praise you with the lyre
for your faithfulness, my God.
—*Psalm 71:9, 21–22, New American Bible*

A sudden illness brings us face-to-face with the feeling of infirmity, something we have traditionally equated with an "older, wiser age." Through our illnesses, we might actually *feel* older at times, especially if we have arthritis or other hallmarks of becoming older. If we have to go on disability and receive Social Security assistance before the age of 65 *and* be on Medicare, well, aren't we just ready to pack it in and go into the "home" already?

Because of our illness, we might be terrified if we think of getting older. If we feel so bad now, what will it be like in five or ten or fifteen years?

Surely those later years won't be "golden" as we'd thought. Unless we're cured, in remission, or recipients of a miraculous healing, our sixties, seventies, and eighties don't look like they're going to be fun at all.

But all around we see people "of a certain age" doing remarkable, life-affirming things. As never before, older men and women are engaging in activities that defy their ages and prove that age, in so many ways, *doesn't matter*. What does matter is the attitude they have, the drive and the determination. The things they accomplish—running marathons, painting masterpieces, writing books, running companies, ministering to others—are not easier because they are older; as anyone ages, they have to face certain health issues.

But the accomplishments have meaning and purpose in a way that those of younger people do not.

What "senior citizens" can do today proves that your life *is* what you make of it.

In the reading from Psalms, David prays that the Lord not cast him aside in his old age. But he doesn't say this just so that he can live longer or just "be" in his older state. No, David wants to be honorable, comforted by God, so that he can praise the Lord with the lyre.

David wants to *do* something in his old age. Just like so many seniors do today.

Examine your fear of getting older.

Do you fear being idle?

Do you fear not having a purpose, a "life beyond merely existing"?

Do you worry that your infirmities will overpower you?

Think of what you do now. Ten years ago, you were that much younger.

Are you any less productive or praiseful than you were then?

If you are, why?

What can you do to change how you are now and plan for how you want to be in the future?

Our lives are constantly moving, growing, aging. We bring all we have learned and experienced with us as we travel along with the Lord. Aging is happening now, just as it will all the rest of our lives, and we have in our power the ability to make of ourselves witnesses, warriors, wonderful people for God and one another.

Our lives are what we make of them, all that we positively can do, now.

And in the future.

Lord, I have feared growing older,
but I know that my life is in your hands.
Let me keep my eyes upon you and my hands busy with
your work.
And let me never be cast aside,
but always find things to do
so that I may praise you and praise you,
my faithful God.

THE GRASS IS GREENER . . .

The people complained against God and Moses, "Why have you brought us up from Egypt to die in this desert, where there is no food or water? We are disgusted with this wretched food!"
— *Numbers 21:5, New American Bible*

The longer you live with a serious illness, the more inclined you might be to become nostalgic for the "good old days" of when you were healthier. Some people, too, forget what it was really like to be healthy and idealize the days gone by, when doctors and medications and pain and discomfort weren't part of their lives.

The Israelites did this as they traveled through the hot desert. Their journey became so unappetizing that even the life-sustaining food they were given wasn't pleasing to them. They longed for the days when they were back in Egypt, almost forgetting that back there, they were subject to Pharaoh as slaves. And they didn't have the patience to sustain them through the desert until they reached the Promised Land—at least, they didn't have it yet.

You might complain to God, "Why did you take away my health? This isn't a *real* life, not like the one I had before." You might think that you had it so much better "back in the good old days." But did you really?

No life, whether healthy or fraught with illness, is devoid of bad moments, difficulty, and pain. To live fully is to experience both the ups and the downs of being human. God doesn't shield us from either of these aspects, nor does he let us "coast" down the middle. He wants us to be engaged in life, to savor its wonder and feel it with heartfelt humanity.

Everyone at some point is led into the desert, into challenge. That is what is happening to you now. Just like the Israelites, no doubt you've wanted to go back to the way things were before your illness. But God is leading you onward, to the Promised Land, and the more you keep this in sight, the more you will be able to cope with your situation now and get from it all the depth and miracles that it can bring.

In this reading from Numbers, there is a curious thing. The Israelites complained that they had no food or water, but in the next breath said they were "disgusted with this wretched food." Clearly they were being given sustenance. And although it was not exactly gourmet fare, it was giving them what they needed to make the journey through the desert to the land God had prepared for them. In your own life, too, the "food" might not be as palatable as it once was, but the Lord gives you exactly what you need. In refining you, in shaping you with his might *and* love, he is giving you the nourishment to fully appreciate and walk into *his* promise to you, which lies on the other side of the desert.

Perhaps at times the grass *does* seem greener as you look at the time when you didn't have your illness. But look before you. The Lord promised a land "flowing with milk and honey" to his Chosen People. To you, he promises all that and more, for you are his child, his beloved for whom he gave his only Son. Understand then that you are going through a process. And the treasures he will give to you upon its completion are

strengthened, made richer by your time now, with every step
you take.

Father, I don't like the things that are happening now
because of my illness.
But help me to be willing to walk through this desert,
for as long as it takes,
and accept what you give me
as the way to arrive at your wonderful Promise
at journey's end.

Prayer for Researchers

The things that mark an apostle—signs, wonders and miracles—
were done among you with great perseverance.
—*2 Corinthians 12:12, New International Version*

Before there can be any new medication, diagnostic tests, or
answers about why people contract certain illnesses, there
must be research. The men and women who carry out this
vital task must be well trained, inquisitive, and extremely patient. They might never win prizes, they might never make a
lot of money (usually, in fact, they don't). They spend countless hours hunched over microscopes or observing chemical
interactions with a focus that doesn't waver, that must not
waver, if they are to find the answers they seek.

In many ways researchers are the unsung heroes and hero-
ines of the world of healthcare. What they do is not glamorous;
working in a laboratory can be a messy, smelly job. It is also
physically demanding; they have to keep sharp eyesight and
endure sore backs and tired minds. But their discoveries can
make huge differences in people's lives. They can find cures,
better treatments, and more information that will help our
doctors make our lives easier.

And, too, researchers can teach us a tremendous lesson!

Probably the greatest asset a researcher can have is that
of perseverance. Experiments must be developed, carried out,

tried, and tried again. Data must be analyzed, gone over thoroughly, and sometimes defended when others question its validity. Studies must be conducted on potentially new medications, and they, too, must be analyzed, presented to review boards, and either accepted or rejected . . . and sometimes conducted all over again.

All of this and the many other processes that go into research take time. A lot of time. There is also a substantial amount of money involved, because all of this work costs millions, billions, and so many projects must be justified financially as well as medically.

All the while, of course, people are suffering from illnesses, seeking answers, and desperate for relief from their suffering. We who have these illnesses sometimes forget that there are lifetimes of work that go into the pills we take, the diagnostic tests we have, and the understanding that we acquire about our conditions. Researchers often dedicate their lives to finding out one fact, uncoding one part of the genetic makeup of an illness, or taking a substance from preliminary possibility to a medication that is put on the market. Naturally, we want quick answers, quick fixes. But often there are none.

We can't just fast forward in time and reap the benefits of researchers' work, skipping the research, development, and approval phases. Better that we stay with them in spirit, keeping them in our prayers. It doesn't matter that we don't know their names or where they live and work. What matters is that we lift up their lives of dedication and discipline to our Lord and ask that they be blessed with wisdom and success in their projects, and that they will conduct their work in a way that is honorable and pleasing to the Lord.

Through the patience that researchers show, we can learn lessons of fortitude and perseverance. And we can understand a little more of how complex the world of medicine is, and how much more we need the Lord in the midst of it.

I do not know the names or recognize the faces
of the researchers who are, this moment,
working on projects that can impact me and others who
suffer from serious illness.
But, Lord, I ask that you bless each one individually.
Help each man and woman researcher to be patient,
full of wisdom,
and conscious of the sacredness of your world.
And help me to appreciate their work and emulate their
perseverance each day.

BEING AN INSTRUMENT
OF PEACE

Let love be sincere, hate what is evil, hold on to what is good; love one another with mutual affection, anticipate one another in showing honor. Do not grow slack in zeal, be fervent in spirit, serve the Lord. Rejoice in hope, endure in affliction, persevere in prayer. Do not be conquered by evil, but conquer evil with good.
—Romans 12:9–12, 21, New American Bible

There were once two men who worked at the same company. Both showed great promise in their work and both were tremendous "team players." When the time came for their boss to decide which one to promote (for there was only one slot open), he gave them each a challenge.

"I want you to each choose a job within this company that you haven't had yet, but that you think will show just how valuable an employee you can be. You will work in the job for two weeks, at the end of which time I'll decide whom I will promote to be my right-hand worker."

The two men agreed this was a brilliant plan. The first man took no time deciding what job he thought would most showcase his talents. He went right up to the boss and said, "I'll just step into that promotion right now, sir. I want to show you how much I can do."

The boss agreed, and the man moved into the office next door.

I'll show him how much I want the job by how much work I can create and how well I supervise others, the man thought. He generated piles of paperwork and nagged his secretary so much that she was in tears by the end of the day. He filled his calendar with lavish business lunches and meetings, and skipped the warehouse foreman's birthday party. The one person he made time for was the boss, and he never failed to "catch" him coming and going to tell him about all the work he was doing and the "great ideas" he had thought of.

Meanwhile, the second man took the job of receptionist. It was perceived as the lowliest job in the company, but the second man enjoyed it because it put him in contact with many people whom he had not met previously, allowed him to see the business "from the ground up," and made him become better versed in the services and products the company produced. Throughout the next two weeks he did not see much of the boss, but that did not bother him much.

I like this place, the second man thought. *And I like the people here. It is a pleasure to work here, no matter what I'm doing.*

At the end of the two weeks, the boss called both men into his office.

"I asked you to each choose a job to perform for two weeks, and now I am going to tell you which of you I will promote."

It should be no surprise that the second man got the job. Even though he had chosen the most lowly job, his sincerity and earnestness were unquestionable. Through his zeal and honor in performing his job well, he learned more than the first man had. And he had enough energy and enthusiasm at the end of the two weeks to keep on doing well—and doing good—in his place of business for some time to come.

* * *

Truly, it does not matter whether we have a responsible job and supervise hundreds of people, or whether we are confined to our homes, sick in bed. What does matter is that we do everything with love, appreciation for others, and a willingness to bring peace to everything and everyone we come in contact with.

Being insincere, haughty, or egotistical takes a lot of extra time and energy. In succumbing to these darker traits, we give in to evil. How much better for us to strip away all artifice and be our genuine, good selves, even through affliction, with an endurance and a spirit that can firmly and finally conquer evil with good.

> *O Lord, make me an instrument of your peace.*
> *Where there is hatred, let me sow your love.*
> *Let me be true to the life you have given me,*
> *and embrace all that is good in it,*
> *so that I may do my job well and find my place*
> *with you.*

THE JOY IN NATURE

The heavens declare the glory of God;
the sky proclaims its builder's craft.
One day to the next conveys that message;
one night to the next imparts the knowledge.
—*Psalm 19:1–3, New American Bible*

Is anything more glorious than a beautiful day? Whether it is thundering dark or brilliantly bright, our Lord's creation of weather, earth, and sky is amazing. God's glory *is* in the stars, the clouds, the sun and the moon. His hand is in the comets and meteors, the storm front and the still, still early morning when the sky is streaked with crimson, pink, and gold.

The creatures of the earth are a wonder to behold, too. Watching a bird soar or a squirrel try to get into a birdfeeder is like having a private show unfolding all for you. The endless stream of butterflies that pass by punctuate our day with awe. The comfort of a beloved pet cannot be overstated.

The Lord has formed this world with sparkling rivers, fathoms-deep oceans, and towering, snowcapped mountains. He has painted it with infinite shades of green and blue, white and brown. He hides treasures within it, precious as gold, silver, and diamonds. And he gives us treasures aboveground in everything he has created.

Whenever I am particularly low, I like to sit by my window

and watch the Lord's nature pass by. Trees sway in the breeze. Seagulls chatter and mince along the ground. Hummingbirds hover over flowers. Roses burst forth with colors and forms so glorious I cannot look away.

Underneath all that the Lord has created, throughout all of his nature, is an emotion that wells up within me whenever I contemplate it. It is joy. And there is, I think, in all of God's nature, the same feeling. After all, the flowers, trees, and birds know no sorrow. They are not frenzied or angry. They are living, fully, in life and in joy. The same is true of the sounds of the world. Sometimes I close my eyes and there, too, feel joy in the music that God plays as the wind blows, the thunder booms, and the grass crunches underfoot. Or I focus on feeling the breeze on my face, the sand in my hand, the moisture in a rain-swept breath . . . in all, there is joy.

Joy is a freeing emotion and one that is important in an illness-shadowed life. To be full of joy is to be praiseful, and to be praiseful is to express our love for God. But too often we equate joy with what someone might give us for a present or tell us as a compliment. Joy is, actually, freeing and free—all around us in the nature created by God! And it is ours for the appreciating, ours for the experiencing.

I have a good friend who has severe, organ-threatening lupus, but who keeps a very positive outlook on life. She tells me, "Even if I feel rotten, I know there's hope and joy. Because the sun comes up every morning and goes down every night and in between, there are all kinds of things to watch and love in the world."

Watching, listening, feeling nature is like witnessing the hand of God work a masterpiece of art. And I feel profoundly glad and grateful that I have this privilege—and joy!

O Lord, sometimes I get so caught up in my narrow world
that I lose sight of the joy that is beyond it.

Please direct my eyes, my ears, indeed all of my senses
to the gift of nature that is all around me.
And let me see the joy
and experience it, more fully
with each delightful miracle that I behold.

LOSING LIBIDO

On my bed at night I sought him
whom my heart loves—
I sought him but I did not find him.
I will rise then and go about the city;
in the streets and crossings I will seek
Him whom my heart loves.
—*The Song of Songs 3:1–2, New American Bible*

Human love in all of its forms is an amazing gift from God. Sadly, in our society we tend to be bombarded by only one aspect of it: sex. On commercials, in advertisements, on talk shows, and in personal conversations, the topic of human, loving relationships swings from "sex" to "SEX!!!" and back again, without much "airtime" devoted to nonintercourse intimacy, empathy, fellowship, mutual respect, and commonality of goals and values.

What must the Lord think of his dear human creation as he observes how crudely his precious gift of human sexuality is being treated?

Moreover, how do we put our own sexuality in a godly perspective when an illness affects our appearance, self-esteem, and drive?

For some people, loss of libido is a devastating side effect to being ill. It can unbalance an otherwise loving relationship between husband and wife, and it can also impact long-term family goals and pregnancy.

But more fundamentally to someone suffering from illness, loss of the feeling of sexuality can shake the foundation of his or her identity as a complete man or woman. And it can bring a profound sadness tied to the loss of physical pleasure and mutual demonstrative affection that two married people naturally enjoy.

When there is an unsettling of balance within someone's life, the evils of the world will try to move in somehow and take over the place where God-centered trust once resided. It is, then, very important to recognize that society's vocal adoration and exploitation of SEX!!! is not to be confused with what we, as Christians, believe.

Sex *is* part of the marital relationship. But a marriage bond that is forged only for physical reasons is doomed to failure. Two people have to have a lot more in common than an active sex life to make a marriage work and thrive, especially today. They need to be tied together through the Holy Spirit, through mutual respect and trust, and through like-minded goals and dreams. They need to really take to heart *all* of the marriage vows and be willing to take one another "in sickness and in health."

The more a couple works together to build the wholeness of their relationship, the stronger they will be in the face of a challenge such as serious illness.

Also, the more the ill spouse is encouraged to develop and appreciate all aspects of his or her being, the easier it will be to weather the disappointment that loss of libido can bring.

For single people, too, it is important to keep in mind that you can be a woman or a man and not have sexual longings. There are so many other things that make us who we are—and so many other gifts that the Lord is willing to give us, if we open our eyes and hearts to accept them.

To be sure, sometimes there is a medical reason for loss of libido, which needs to be addressed by qualified doctors. But whether there is or is not a medical basis for the loss of feeling sexually charged, there is an underlying truth:

If you look for other ways to express your love with your husband or wife and build your marriage into a firm, God-centered house, and if you recognize that you are a unique, complex man or woman in the eyes of the Lord, your life will be more deeply satisfying than you ever thought possible.

O Lord, I am afraid that losing my libido might
ruin my life.
I want to be a good spouse, and I want to be able
to appreciate
my body and being as you have created them.
Please help me see beyond my disappointment
and worry
and find a deeper existence,
a more whole life,
with you as my guide and Savior.

INFERTILITY

But the LORD said to Abraham: "Why did Sarah laugh and say,
'Shall I really bear a child, old as I am?' Is anything too marvelous
for the LORD to do?"
— *Genesis 18:13–14, New American Bible*

I pestered my parents for almost five years to give me a baby
brother. From my childish perspective, nothing should have
been easier. After all, my playmates had brothers and sisters,
and my aunts and uncles seemed to add to their families each
year. So I nagged and pleaded and finally, one glorious day, we
went to an adoption agency and brought home a baby boy.

From the day he arrived in our house, I loved him as completely as any sibling loves another. It didn't matter that he
wasn't a "real" brother, born from my mother. All that mattered was that I finally had "my baby brother." We played, argued, fought, and planned countless pranks . . . all like regular
siblings do. Nothing was more natural to me than having this
rambunctious boy as my brother.

As I got older, however, I learned that there are some people who don't view an adopted boy or girl as a "true" member
of the family. Some men I have spoken with have even insisted
that they could never accept a child into their home if it
weren't "really" theirs. And through the years I have heard stories of couples who went to great lengths, emotionally, physi-

149

cally, and financially, to overcome their infertility rather than adopt a child.

I understand the deep need to have children and respect the desire to nurture the next generation. And I certainly sympathize deeply with couples who cannot conceive. But through my own experience of having an adoptive brother, I also wonder if they know what they are missing. There are after all many babies in this world who need good, loving homes. There are many children, too, who have outgrown diapers but are in no less need of finding a nurturing family environment to develop and grow in. And while adoptive children might not share a couple's genetic makeup, can we really say that any other human being "belongs to us" when we know that each person ultimately belongs to the Lord?

Infertility due to an illness or as the result of prescribed treatments, medications, or surgery can be completely devastating to a couple. It can also negatively affect new relationships, if one person involved wants to have children and the other cannot. But there are ways to be a parent and not bear children of your own. And there are so many needy children yearning for the opportunity to be called "daughter" or "son."

In the reading from Genesis, clearly Sarah has moved beyond disappointment at not being able to bear children and is openly laughing when she hears that God has promised her and her husband Abraham a son. Her acceptance of her condition shows how far she has come, and also how much more miraculous God's power can be. And ultimately, her deepest wish is fulfilled and she does bear a son, just as the Lord promised.

We do not know the mind of the Lord. We cannot say that, if we are infertile today, we will always be so. But we can accept our condition now and act to do the Lord's bidding. If it is his will that we be parents, he will ordain it. If it is his will that we adopt, he will ready our hearts and homes and make that happen, too. Whichever way he chooses to bring us into the lives of the next generation, we can be assured that his love will spill over into our hearts, for nothing is "too marvelous" for the Lord.

O Lord, I want to be a parent,
but I do not know how it is to happen.
Let me put all my trust, all my faith in you.
Prepare in me a heart full of love,
for the child you may one day entrust with me.

BECOMING ADDICTED TO PRESCRIPTION MEDICATION

Save me, God,
for the waters have reached my neck.
—*Psalm 69:1, New American Bible*

You think the pills you hold in your hand will bring you relief from your pain. But over time, one pill seems not enough. So you take two. Then three. Then four. And even that might not be enough. Before you can stop yourself, what began as a simple way to sleep at night or bend or walk without excruciating pain becomes an obsession. You want more pills. You *need* more pills. And you start to look for illegal ways to obtain them.

Your illness takes a backseat to your need for more pills. Your family takes a backseat, too, as does your job and any outside interests.

You are drowning. Drowning in addiction to prescription medication.

You never meant for this to happen.

But it does.

. . .

When we take medications to alleviate our suffering, we usually do not think that they will do more harm than good. But unfortunately, many of the prescription medicines our doctors prescribe for us can have dangerous ramifications. Instead of helping us then, these medicines for pain and other symptoms or conditions can take us into the dark, deep world of addiction. Law-abiding individuals might start forging prescriptions to get more pills. Otherwise upstanding individuals might steal from friends and relatives.

As the addiction gets more entrenched within the patient's psyche, everything else, including relationships, work, even the person's health, will begin to suffer. One person formerly addicted to pain medication told me that those days of drug dependence were "like living in hell where nothing else mattered but getting more and more pills."

Are you afraid you are becoming addicted to the medication you are taking now?

Do you fear you might already be addicted?

Until fairly recently, when we heard the word "addict," we thought only of those who were addicted to alcohol, illegal drugs, gambling, or other entities. We might have associated moral decline with these conditions and people and judged them accordingly. Now, however, the medical community is beginning to publicly acknowledge and provide information and hope for those patients who have become addicted to prescription medicines, particularly painkillers. Powerful narcotics and other drugs have been shown to have addictive properties and interactions that can render otherwise law-abiding people "hooked." Social stigmas against people addicted to prescription medicines are gradually fading in light of the new scientific understanding of what happens to some people who take certain drugs. There are now treatment programs, follow-ups, and counseling specifically aimed at these addicts and their loved ones.

Yes, there is hope for anyone who feels that the "waters have reached my neck."

But the first step in getting help and being rescued from the rising waters of addiction is the personal responsibility of the addict.

You need to take a strong, honest look at your behavior and realize that you have a serious, life-altering and perhaps life-threatening problem.

This can be a very sobering experience. Suddenly your addiction and perhaps illegal activities seem to crash down upon your pain-wracked shoulders. Perhaps you have lost your marriage, your house, your children. Perhaps you have ended up on the streets, doing things that you never in a million years thought you would do to simply survive. Perhaps you have forgotten that God still loves you and wants what is best for you.

Your despair becomes overwhelming.

How, you wonder, *will I get out of this alive?*

Throughout Scripture there is evidence of God's might and constancy. When all forsake you, God never will. Now more than ever, you need to trust and believe in him, so present in verse and truth. With him as your partner, you can begin to look honestly at your life. And with each day, each step forward, you can start to feel more in control of the seemingly uncontrollable.

Admitting you have an addiction is not easy, nor is it a quick fix. But it is the first, crucial step toward becoming whole again.

And God is with you now and always.

O Lord, with each new day, help me to be strong and
continue to trust you.

Peace in the Storm

Bring into my eyes and heart
an honesty that sees my true situation
and finds support in your goodness and guidance.
Let me see release from my addiction
and a renewed joy in living from this day forward.

Changing Your Attitude
toward Your Life

All the days of the oppressed are wretched,
but the cheerful heart has a continual feast.
—*Proverbs 15:15, New International Version*

"Oh, you have lupus?" someone said to me. "All you have to do is have a positive attitude. Then everything will be just fine."

"No," said someone else. "Lupus is horrible. You'll never have a life. You might as well face it now rather than be even more disappointed later."

What's a newly diagnosed "lupie" to believe?

As I've found out, there's a grain of truth in both of the attitudes toward serious illness. Even with a very positive attitude, I've still suffered from horrible symptoms, worsening conditions, medication side effects, new diseases . . . everything is *not* fine! But then, everything is not so bad, either. Being ill, I've been able to reach a depth of faith and understanding that I never would have arrived at had I always been healthy. And I've been able to get to know incredible people who never would have crossed my path had I not traveled this way.

Indeed, it is through having a positive attitude while acknowledging and accepting hardship that I've been able to cope fairly well with my disease—and any other "curveball" that comes along. It isn't that I'm not saddened, angered, or frustrated by my illness, and it certainly isn't that I have no fear of becoming more ill. No, I own up to all of these very human, very real emotions. But what I've learned to do is face the challenges and ask God and myself, "Now, what am I going to *do* about them?"

When you don't feel well, it is very easy to be oppressed by illness, to be a victim to pain, infection, financial overload, and a life spiraling downhill. Sometimes you don't have the energy or strength to fight all of the negative emotions that can assail you and wear you down. But if you look upon these stumbling blocks as part of a larger whole, you will see that they are not so insurmountable that the Lord can't help you overcome them. And, through prayer and in faith, you can find ways to make the most of them, even turn them around so that you have more control over your life, not less.

Yes, you *can* go from being a victim of serious illness to being in charge.

You can control what you eat, how you monitor your health, how you work with your doctors.

You can find support groups, loving friends and family members, and new activities to make up for what you cannot do.

You can be a voice for your illness and support funding for research and patient information.

You can deepen in faith, not fall away from it, and you can witness to others and be a true light for the darkness that falls around so many.

You can be a brilliant soldier for the Lord, even if you are bedridden!

You can see the positive in the negative—and make it work for the Kingdom of God!

The rewards of doing this are certainly in heaven, but they are also here on earth. How splendid it is to have a purpose, to know that you are useful and vibrantly alive. How marvelous it is to enjoy close relationships and to know that you are genuinely loved, and loving in return.

How fantastic to wake up each day with a goal in mind—and see it come to fruition!

You don't have to make changes in what you do and think all at once. But bit by bit, day by day, you will be amazed at the miracles that happen because you are changing your attitude toward your life with illness.

God's blessings are clearly upon me, and for that I praise him and give him all the glory.

If you do not feel this way now, you will be able to. All it takes is a little "change of attitude" to make a huge, life-affirming difference!

O Lord, I do not want to be the victim of my illness,
but rather I want to use it for your glory and good.
Help me find ways to take charge of it,
to change my sadness to determination and joy,
and let me be a light for others, and a bringer
of the gladdest of tidings!

REJOICING IN THE HAPPINESS
OF OTHERS

"A cheerful look brings joy to the heart,
good news makes for good health."
—*Proverbs 15:30, New Living Translation*

How much good news have you heard today? A lot? A little? Enough?

So much of our lives is taken up with bad world news or difficult personal situations that it can seem as if all of the good news is crowded out or nonexistent. But hearing of happy events and being able to rejoice in them with others is such a wonderful, uplifting part of living that we shouldn't let the negative side of life overshadow them. Rather, we should seek them!

With a serious illness, it can be much more difficult to get out and attend weddings, parties, or other joyful events with friends and family. It can also be costly if travel, gifts, and lodging are involved. But there are other ways to express joy at the good fortune of others, and ways that you can still be a part of the happiness in their lives. Crafting your own cards and gifts is one way of making your expression personal and meaningful. So, too, is making a long long-distance phone call to a friend or relative who's too far away to visit with in person.

Being of cheerful heart yourself will invite others to see the positive side of their lives and can foster more uplifting conversations, especially if you accompany your lightened emotions with laughter and smiles. Opening your eyes and heart to stories of human triumph and heroism can help balance the other, more somber stories that you hear—and feed your soul with more of God's glory.

Simple happiness is as valid and important as great milestones in anyone's life; finding those smaller, brighter joys is part of the "good news" that makes for "good health." Sharing a beautiful day or a funny cartoon with a loved one, applauding a friend's new hairstyle, or giving someone a compliment on his or her strength of character or courage—all of these are ways to rejoice in the happiness of others and bring that "good medicine" into your life of chronic illness.

It is easy to fall prey to jealousy when we are seriously ill. We might resent others' good health or their ability to do things we no longer can. We also might detest the fact that we have to spend our money on medication instead of vacations or wear last year's clothing instead of buying a new wardrobe. The sense of the world moving on without us can create a deep sense of betrayal, and envy, too.

Of all the negative emotions, jealousy can eat away at us longest and most profoundly, and cause a bitterness that can undermine our search for strong faith and God's abiding comfort. The farther we go from God's love, the farther we sink into a morass of unhappiness, creating a cycle that pulls us downward at a time when we should most want to be striving *up*ward.

We are eager for health, eager for what is good and just. So we combat our jealousy by acknowledging that we *are* precious children of the Lord. We *do* have wonderful gifts in our lives, things that we can do and have that are individual to us. And we want to share our happiness with others, just as much as we want to share theirs.

In a world of darkness, we are called to be light. In a tasteless world, we are called to bring delicious flavor. In rejoicing in the happiness of others, we continue our witness in the world and put the jealousy in our hearts to rest, forever standing on God's promises for us and filling our hearts with joy that will make for good health, for good wholeness, for all concerned.

O Lord, still the jealousy in my heart
and put in it instead a genuine happiness for others
who are celebrating something wonderful.
Let me be cheerful for them, because of them,
and let me show that Christian love and charity
transcend all human failings.

OVERLOADED WITH
FINANCIAL WORRY

"If God so clothes the grass of the field, which grows today and is thrown into the oven tomorrow, will he not much more provide for you? . . . So do not worry and say, 'What are we to eat?' or 'What are we to drink?' or 'What are we to wear?' Your heavenly Father knows you need them all."
—*Matthew 6:30–32, New American Bible*

A serious illness can be very expensive. On top of your insurance premiums (if you have insurance) is a staggering world of co-pays, medication costs, and lost wages from missed work. You might have to completely redesign your living space to accommodate your physical needs. You might have to buy a new wardrobe or purchase other health aids that are necessities in your new life with illness.

Along with these new expenses, your usual day-to-day costs might increase. Food, shelter, transportation can be extremely expensive, and if you are also responsible for providing for a family, you can be overloaded with financial worries. These worries become stresses. Stresses can aggravate health conditions, potentially creating more medical problems. Your healthcare costs might rise even more.

But in the midst of this seemingly endless cycle, the Lord tells us to not worry! He knows what we need. He will not forsake us.

"If God so clothes the grass of the field, which grows today and is thrown into the oven tomorrow, will he not much more provide for you?"

Yes, we need to have faith that the Lord will provide. But it's hard to believe that he'll just drop a big check on our doorstep each month to cover the expenses of all our bills!

Involving the Lord in our lives is a very proactive thing. We need to participate in his creation and be instruments of his good works. Thus, lifting our financial concerns to the Lord is the first step in allowing him to work in our lives. We need to be receptive to his kindness, open to his generosity. If we just sit by and expect him to send manna from heaven, we might be waiting a long time.

Because we feel we are needy is no reason to ignore the needs of others. We also need to be active in the lives of others, providing for them when called upon just as they provide for us when we need it. In doing this we are full participants in the Lord's creation and full members of the body of Christ.

Through our prayer and introspection, God will reveal his way and his will for us. We might not need all that we think we need. We might be able to substitute some products for others. We might discover alternative ways of shopping, working, or providing for our family that are more aligned with what he wants for us and with what we truly need. Taking to heart the phrase "You can't take it with you" will help differentiate what are essential expenses and what things are extraneous, even frivolous. And humbling ourselves to live in a more Christlike manner will take away our material desires and put in their place hearts of wholesome gladness.

Above all, we have to trust that as long as we act in a way

that is pleasing to the Lord, we will not go hungry, we will have shelter, we will be taken care of. This is the Lord's promise to us. How wonderful is the Lord!

> *O Lord, the financial aspect of my illness is*
> *overwhelming.*
> *Help me put all my money worries into perspective.*
> *Let me know how to spend and save wisely,*
> *to do what is necessary to allow you to work through me*
> *and keep my hope and trust in you*
> *more true than any desire for material gain or goods.*

FEAR OF PASSING YOUR ILLNESS ALONG TO YOUR CHILD

> May the LORD bless you from Zion,
> all the days of your life.
> That you may share Jerusalem's joy
> and live to see your children's children.
> Peace upon Israel!
> —*Psalm 128:5–6, New American Bible*

Sometimes scientists can determine what causes an illness, but sometimes they cannot. It is frustrating to think that you might not be able to pinpoint the reason for your developing condition. It can be frightening to think that what you have might be passed along to your children. Frightening, yes, and even terrifying.

Becoming a parent brings with it certain responsibilities, among which is wanting and providing the very best environment for your child. This includes making sure your child is safe, secure, and healthy. But what if you have an illness that might have a genetic component? What if there is a possibility that you could pass your illness along to your child?

In our very scientific world, there could be statistics and even tests that might tell you what the chances are of your child having or developing the same illness you have. Some diseases have been definitively linked to genetics and might be identifiable even before conception, given the availability of tests for you and your spouse. But even the best of science does not take into account the power of our Lord and the magnitude of his involvement in our lives and the lives of our children. Sometimes, even when a couple does not plan to have a child, they conceive—more proof that God's will surpasses all human (and scientific) understanding!

There might be a high statistical probability that your child will develop your illness, but this doesn't account for God's will in the matter. The same Lord who can move mountains can protect your child from illness. It is part of our faith, part of our trust, that his will can be greater than anything under heaven or on earth.

On the other hand, if it is God's will that you have a child and that child carries the illness you have, the Lord has a purpose there, too. For, as you know from your own experience with serious illness, there is much joy and much learning to be found in suffering, and much of God's glory to be experienced.

Whether your child does or does not develop your illness, the Lord will provide you with the tools and grace to be a good parent and a nurturing witness. And he will heap upon you both his gracious mercy and his love. He will never forsake you or your child, and he will make a way for you, even through the darkest desert.

In this reading from Psalms, God's blessing is clear: "Peace be upon you, and may you 'share Jerusalem's joy and live to see your children's children.'" Even though our fear of passing along illness is human, it pales when we think of this powerful blessing and what it means to our lives. If peace is upon us, there is no room for fear. If we are to share joy, then certainly the gift of a dear child will be a mighty happiness and a manifestation of God's love. And if the Lord wishes us to live to see our children's children, he will find a way for that to happen in spite of any scientific probability to the contrary.

O Lord, I stand before you humbled and mindful of
your power over my life
and the practice and belief of science.
Please help me do what you will in parenthood
and in nurturing my children,
and approach their lives, as I do my life,
in full presence of your power, grace, and love.

A Bad Reaction to Medication

The LORD is my shepherd;
there is nothing I lack.
In green pastures, you let me graze;
to safe waters you lead me;
you restore my strength.
—*Psalm 23:1–2, New American Bible*

One night not long ago, I took a new kind of medication that was supposed to help one of my very severe lupus symptoms. I had read all the accompanying literature and knew that there could be side effects, but it wasn't until late into the night that I felt the full force of what those effects were. I had the worst nightmares I've ever had, one after the other, and finally woke in the still of the night shaking from anxiety and sure that some horrible monster was about to strike.

In the midst of this awful experience, however, I also knew that what I was going through was due to the new medication (which I then and there promised never to take again). While my mind was still reeling from the nightmares and anxiety, I recited this reading from Psalms over and over until finally I fell asleep. This time I had no nightmares, and although I awakened exhausted and weak, I knew that my "dark night of the medication" had passed. I knew that the reading from

Psalms had been my antidote against the horrors that assailed me—and I praised God for bringing me through!

As a responsible patient, you know how important it is to be fully informed about any medication you take. Your doctor and your pharmacist are important resources for information about side effects and medication interactions. But even in the most careful of situations, bad reactions can occur. Of course, you need to address these quickly, even seeking emergency medical treatment if necessary. But along with the practical actions you should take, you also can turn to Scripture and prayer to ease your anxiety and bring you through the experience in peace.

I have memorized this reading from Psalms, as I am sure many Christians (and even non-Christians) have. I keep it close to my heart and turn to it as often as I need to to burn it like a brand upon my soul and let its full impact be felt in every cell of my body and being. I know that the Lord led me through that night when I had the horrible reaction to my medication, and I also know that he will lead me through to "safe waters" every time I call upon him.

This knowledge is powerful medicine and is available to us for the asking. We lack nothing with the Lord guiding us. And even if we are buffeted by medication side effects, we can make it through to safety *and* have our strength restored by the Lord.

Know this reading from Psalms. *Believe* that the Lord is your shepherd.

Always. Everywhere.

Lord Jesus, be my shepherd.
When I have a bad reaction to medication,
bring me to the proper medical treatment
and calm my troubled soul.
Restore my strength, and bring me to the safe waters
where you are my rock and my deliverer.

What Does the Rainbow Mean to You?

God added: "This is the sign that I am giving for all ages to come,
of the covenant between me and you and every living creature with
you: I set my bow in the clouds to serve as a sign of the covenant
between me and the earth. When I bring clouds over the earth, and
the bow appears in the clouds, I will recall the covenant I have made
between me and you and all living things so that the waters shall
never again become a flood to destroy all mortal beings."
—*Genesis 9:12–15, New American Bible*

To the Israelites, the rainbow was the sign of God's covenant with them. After the flood, God promised he would
never again bring such waters to "destroy all mortal beings."
And in doing so, he brought an abiding hope in the future that
his Chosen People had not felt before. If there was to be no
earth-engulfing flood again, then there was hope of tomorrow.
There was a promise of days, weeks, years to come. And there
was the knowledge that life would continue for generations.

Far from being a distant memory, the promise of the rainbow is still a vibrant presence today. Knowing as we do that
centuries have passed since Noah's time, we are aware that the
Lord has kept his covenant and word—no flood has since cov-

ered all the reaches of the earth. This multicolored sign arcing over the sky has decorated the world and rested in the hearts of all believers who have gone before us.

And it is relevant for we who live now.

What does this rainbow mean to you today?

Have you confined its meaning to the pages of your Bible, or have you truly taken it into all aspects of your life?

Is the rainbow a meteorological phenomenon that spans the skies after a storm, or is it something active each moment of the day?

Now, more than ever, when you are suffering from a serious illness and your life seems to be in turmoil, you need the constant reassurance that God's covenant of sustenance and salvation will be with you through it all. In this context, the rainbow takes on a greater meaning than a mere natural occurrence. It comes alive and expands. It brings hope.

The rainbow can be found in all things that bring you comfort and deeper faith in God's promises. From a baby's smile to the opening of the morning flowers to the brilliant scarlet of a sunset, the rainbow is present, and with it, God's abiding covenant.

In illness, too, the rainbow is present. It is in the expertise of the medical professionals who treat us, the researchers who hunt for cures, the medication that we take each day that gives us more time and more relief.

Truly, the more you recognize the rainbow's message in things around you, the more you will feel God's presence, power, compassion, and hope.

I keep a picture of a rainbow in my kitchen. It is a snapshot that I took after rains drenched the area and dark clouds hovered in the sky. It reminds me of the presence of God in my neighborhood, on my street, and of the beauty that lives in spite of the storm. It also helps me remember to look for the rainbow in every hardship, in every day. In doing this, I am filled with hope. My own storms become finite, not endless. And my faith is magnified.

God has never taken back his covenant. He hasn't reneged on his promise to the Israelites. In fact, he expanded upon this divine commission by giving us the gift of his only Son Jesus Christ and bringing us fully into his Salvation.

The rainbow, for us, is more than an arc of colors in the sky. We can find the rainbow all around us and within us, in nature and in ourselves. It is the deep, abiding promise of God to us that, no matter the trouble or pain, he sustains us.

He does not destroy.

He saves.

O Lord, in my suffering, let me remember
your promise.
Help me to see your rainbow
emblazoned upon the sky and in my heart.
And let its promise be with me and sustain me
through all storms,
for all of my days.

BEING TRULY RESTFUL

By the seventh day God had finished the work he had been doing;
so on the seventh day he rested from all his work. And God blessed
the seventh day and made it holy, because on it he rested from all
the work of creating that he had done.

—*Genesis 2:2–3, New International Version*

Resting, truly resting, is an art that is in danger of disappearing in today's world. If we are to leave on vacation,
we have to scramble to get "everything done" before we go,
and sometimes we take work with us. If we decide to have a
"restful" night at home, we might fill it with television, reading, or picking up around the house. If we do decide to "do
nothing," we might become very anxious and nervous, as if
there's something wrong with "just being." And as for keeping
a whole day of the week restful—well, that seems almost impossible!

God's example, as described in Genesis, is very enlighten-
ing. Not only did the Lord create the world, but he took a
whole day off afterward! And not only did he make that day
one of rest, he also "made it holy."

How different would our restful time be if we thought of
it as "holy"? How much easier would it be to take a whole day
off each week if we kept in mind that it was to be lifted up to
the Lord?

I have heard some lupus patients say that when they go on vacation, "lupus takes a vacation, too." Of course, this isn't true; chronic illness doesn't go away simply because we have travel plans! But this concept of taking a break from our illness is useful, if only to help us recoup our energies and prepare for the days when it will take the forefront of our activity and attention. Truly, we *need* downtime, restful time, when we can be still and let the Lord revive our weary bodies and hearts.

We need to take our cue from God, who rested on the seventh day and kept it holy. We need to be truly restful, on a regular basis.

At first the thought of taking a whole day off might seem like an impractical aspiration. If you are running a household, working a time-consuming job, or parenting children, you might think that your time is uncontrollable. But, as with everything, the Lord knows what you need.

In prayer, meditate on his desire for you to have restful time as well as busy time. Pray for guidance to know when you can make "holy" time—that is, time when you can rest from all of your work and just "be" with the Lord. Maybe it isn't an entire day at first; perhaps it is an hour or two a week. Above all, it is important that you not be stressed about taking this time. It is holy time, dedicated time, *restful* time. No television. No chores. No distractions. Just time with the Lord *after* all of your work.

In today's world, time is something that should be filled with other things. By setting the example of taking time to rest for a full day, the Lord is showing us that time is also something to be made holy by itself. Just as we smell a flower or feel sand between our toes, time is to be enjoyed for what it is, a gift and opportunity to rest as well as to work.

Creating the world is an awesome accomplishment, and how we praise the Lord for it! How wonderful, too, that God has given us his example of resting on the seventh day, so that we might see that, just as important as our work is, so too is making some time holy, restful, and blessed.

O Lord, I fill my days with activities and thoughts
that take me far from being truly restful.
But let me learn from your example of resting on the
seventh day,
and help me to find time, to make it holy,
devoid of work, but full of your blessing
of refreshment and rejuvenation.

Complying with Prescribed Medical Treatment

> Blessed is the man who perseveres in temptation, for when he has been proven he will receive the crown of life that [the Lord] promised to those who love him.
>
> —*James 1:12, New American Bible*

At some point during treatment for your illness, you might become tempted to stop taking your medication or continuing under your doctor's care. Perhaps your symptoms are not lessening, despite all that your doctor is prescribing, or perhaps you have heard of other ways to combat your illness that aren't in keeping with "traditional" medicine. Perhaps, too, you are getting impatient with being ill and somehow hope that by stopping your medication or cutting back on it, you won't be sick any longer.

Thinking of going off of your medication is in part tied in with denial. Some medication works so subtly that you might think it's not doing any good, and you could start wondering if it will make any difference if you continue taking it or not. You might even begin to doubt that you're sick at all, not realizing that the medication *is* working to keep you from becoming more ill.

Another aspect of being tempted to go off of your current

treatment comes from outside forces: well-meaning friends or others who insist they know better than your doctor what is right for you. Some people might say that they "don't believe in taking all that medication," or others will tout the latest "alternative" treatment instead of what you're doing. You might feel swayed by them, persuaded that they *do* know better.

Still another reason for not complying with your prescribed medical treatment is your own procrastination, laziness, or lack of consistency.

There are so many reasons why we might be tempted to go off of our meds or stop seeing our doctors!

But in light of all of these reasons and others we might have, we have to stand firm. We have to believe in the Lord's guidance, stay in his wisdom, and do what is ultimately the *right* thing, no matter what others might say.

In prayerful silence, explore the reasons why you want to stop taking your medication. Away from distractions or others who would persuade you otherwise, ask God to help you sort out why it is you don't want to see your doctor anymore. Face reality with the Lord by your side, and he will give you the courage and stamina to stay the course, no matter the obstacles.

Treating serious illness today is a complex and very amazing thing. Doctors spend years in study and practice to learn the intricacies of their chosen field. We patients have to understand that there will be some things we *don't* understand, and we must have some faith and trust that our doctors do know more than we do. For example, some medications are most effective when they build up in the system, and others must be tapered in dosage before going off of them. It is never a good idea to stop taking your medication "cold turkey" without your doctor's approval, just as it is never a good idea to stop seeing your doctor if you have an ongoing illness.

The temptation might be there, inside of you and coming

at you from other sources, to fall away from your prescribed medical treatment. But if you are relying on the Lord for guidance and you have a medical team that is competent and well versed in your condition, you need to cultivate trust.

Keep close to the Lord in prayer that he is leading you on the right path in handling your illness, as in all matters in our lives.

View temptation as a challenge, like so many others when you have a serious illness, and make overcoming it a victory.

Father in heaven, help me to be strong, to see my
treatment through
even when the time gets long and my resolve falters.
Let me build faith and trust in my doctors and the
treatment they prescribe
and give them the time they need to work.
Let me overcome temptation
and rise to victory, strengthened and made more whole.

MEMBER OF A REMARKABLE COMMUNITY

Praise be to the God and Father of our Lord Jesus Christ, the Father of compassion and the God of all comfort, who comforts us in all our troubles, so that we can comfort those in any trouble with the comfort we ourselves have received from God.

—2 Corinthians 1:3–4, New International Version

In my life with lupus, I have met many remarkable men and women who share my disease and experience many of the same things I do. I am truly grateful to be part of this community. Yes, grateful and humbled. For there is nothing more incredible or inspiring than the people who take their adversity of ill health and turn it into a positive, shining witness for the Lord. Many times, I feel that I can barely live up to the examples of courage all around me.

You, too, are a person of courage by the very nature of the health challenges you are facing. And you are also part of the remarkable community of like-sufferers. Each day the pain, fear, and hope you experience are also punctuating the lives of other men and women. Each day, too, you are being joined in prayer by them the world over. Why, at this very minute, someone might be reading the very same page that you are in this book!

Besides being tied together by illness, you are also united with your fellow sufferers in compassion and understanding. Who better to know what you're going through than someone on a similar path? This is why support groups are such sources of strength and guidance; we can learn so much from each other, and feel tremendous kinship and sustenance, too.

Knowing that there are others who share your illness makes your walk less lonely. Even though you don't know everyone who has diabetes or cancer, muscular dystrophy or chronic fatigue syndrome, you can be assured that your experience is shared and your life is not being lived in a vacuum. And with the resources available to us today through organizations and on the Internet, there are many places where we can "meet," share our stories, and feel more a part of a vibrant whole.

Through your faith, your place in the body of Christ is established. This sharing is an amazing affirmation of God's gathering his children from all the corners of the earth. How wonderful, too, is his gift of a community of fellow travelers along the road of serious illness. Although this is a group we never thought we would want to be part of, now that we are members, we are firsthand witnesses to the many acts of courage and resilience demonstrated by these remarkable men and women. We reap benefits from our membership that cannot be quantified, or perhaps even explained to people outside our realm of experience. But we know that we are made better and more hopeful through this strong brotherhood with others who suffer as we do.

What a fellowship we enjoy when we suffer from serious illness! How wonderful is the knowledge that there are many others like us all around the world and that we are not alone. Rather, we are united with them through prayer, like experience, and God's community.

Praise be to the Lord!

Father in heaven, I never thought I'd be grateful
to be ill,
but in bringing me this burden, you have also
introduced me
to many remarkable men and women of faith
who share my affliction.
Thank you for introducing me to this
amazing community,
in which I am made strong and through which
I can grow
into a more whole person.

BRAIN FOG

Have mercy on me, O God, have mercy.
I look to you for protection.
I will hide beneath the shadow of your wings
until this violent storm is past.
—*Psalm 57:1, New Living Translation*

Y ou are in a balloon filled with thick, foggy air. You reach
out but cannot connect with the world around you, nor
are your thoughts clear. Rather, everything is tinged with a
haze that prevents you from looking ahead or backward. You
struggle to think of words and form sentences. When you do
speak, your voice sounds to you as though it is coming from
far away. Your actions seem heavy and ineffective. Whether lying down or standing, your world is lethargic, your brain is
moving in slow motion.

To many of us with lupus, or people with chronic fatigue
syndrome, fibromyalgia, or other like illnesses, the above description outlines the phenomenon known as "brain fog." It is
one of the most frustrating aspects of living with these conditions because it strikes at the very center of our thought
processes and lives. Without being able to think clearly, we feel
vulnerable and afraid. At the very least, we find ourselves apol-
ogizing for our memory lapses and halfheartedly laughing

at our perceived "airhead-like" way of communicating. But when the brain fog is really bad and lasts for days, we might become increasingly terrified that it is going to be permanent, that we'll lose what precious little ability we have to engage ourselves in the world.

Although there are some medical treatments for certain kinds of brain fog, for some people this condition is a constant and worsening struggle. For one thing, we *know* we are being gripped by an inability to be connected with ourselves and the world around us. For another, because it is an "invisible" ailment, it might be perceived by some people to be "merely" a function of being stressed or getting older. With each successive episode we might experience more despair, worrying about becoming senile or falling victim to a kind of reverse-adulthood where we cannot even speak coherently.

When I first experienced brain fog, I knew it was something not "normal" for me. No amount of stress or activity had ever brought about the deep sense of disconnectedness that I felt. Finally, after undergoing some tests and scans, I discovered that there was an underlying physical reason for my cognitive problem. But I can't say that this diminished my anxiety over it. Rather, knowing that there was proof of it on paper somehow made me more fearful that it was the "beginning of the end."

It wasn't until I began to pray the above Psalm that my worry started to dissipate. Being caught up in brain fog is very much like "hiding" from the world; how much more comforting to "hide beneath the shadow" of the Lord's wings? When brain fog is particularly bad, I cannot articulate all the prayers and praise that are in my heart; asking for mercy and looking to God for protection are perfect ways of ridding myself of the guilt of not being "fully functional" while at the same time finding refuge until "this violent storm is past."

Thankfully, each time I've lifted up my fears and fog to the Lord, he has taken them away. Not overnight, sometimes, but eventually. In this, as in all things, I'm learning to trust him.

More important, I'm learning to bring him into my life with illness, no matter how small or large the health issues seem to be. Having him beside me and around me gives me security for the times when I am weakest, and calm for the times when the fog is so thick I can't navigate.

In truth, he is the lighthouse, shining clearly through the misty night sea.

O Lord, I am sorry that sometimes I can't articulate
my prayers and praise to you as clearly as I would like.
But even more, I am grateful that you are there,
even in my weakness.
And you give me no cause to fear, but rather to rejoice
that you are
my light and my refuge.

WHEN NO ONE CAN FIND WHAT'S WRONG

My heart is in anguish within me,
the terrors of death assail me.
Fear and trembling have beset me;
horror has overwhelmed me.
I said, "Oh, that I had the wings of a dove!
I would fly away and be at rest."
—*Psalm 55:4–6, New International Version*

With all of the diagnostic procedures available to medical professionals, you would think that all ailments could be diagnosed, or at least identified. Sometimes, however, all of the blood tests and procedures cannot find out what is physically wrong. At these times, not knowing can be much worse than having a definite diagnosis. How the mind can race at all the options when none are ruled out! If your doctor says, "There's something wrong, but we can't yet pinpoint what it is," you might immediately begin thinking of every horror imaginable, even unto death. And you might, as in this reading from Psalms, plead with the Lord, declaring that you would rather have "the wings of a dove" to "fly away and be at rest."

Symptoms can become amplified in the face of the unknown. Pain can become more acute. Every twinge or tremor can seem like a signal that something else is going wrong. You might come to feel as though you are covered by a blanket of illness so thick and impenetrable that no one will ever know what it is or how to treat it.

Your life might seem like an endless spiral downward into a murky, swirling mess.

But there is One who knows all, and he is the Lord. Even if human understanding is limited, his power of knowledge is without bounds. He knows how you suffer, but he also knows that there is a reason for it. In time and with patience, he will reveal all you and your doctors need to know to handle your condition. This is a lifeline, and you need to cling to it as you go from doctor to doctor and through test upon test. It is a truth that rests in our faith and a foundation upon which we can begin to build hope for what is going on in our lives and in the future.

You need strength to be able to seek a diagnosis, to get to the bottom of why you feel the way you do.

The Lord can give you that strength, all that you require.

If, then, you cling to the lifeline thrown to you by our Lord and trust in his Word, you will know that each step you take is pulling you farther away from the "swirling mess" toward knowledge and light. Each test brings you one bit closer to diagnosis. Each doctor's appointment brings you that much closer to treatment. By staying firm with the Lord, you will be able to insist upon additional tests if need be, or second opinions. You will be able to hear his voice within you and speak words that bring you closer and finally up to your diagnosis and treatment.

As children of the Lord, we are hopeful believers that he wants what is best for us. We also know that his time is not necessarily our time. Although it might take more days, weeks, or months to get a firm diagnosis for our illness, it is his will that eventually the best will be done for us. Trusting in this and clinging to his lifeline will lead us away from our fears and overactive imaginations and into a process of positive action and triumph.

O Lord, although no mortal can tell what is wrong,
I know that you know.
Help me to increase my trust in you
that your time is good and your will is supreme.
And give me the words and actions to lead me to my diagnosis,
to what is best in your eyes and in your way.

KEEPING HOPE IN THE HOSPITAL

But the LORD sent a large fish, that swallowed Jonah; and he remained in the belly of the fish three days and three nights. From the
belly of the fish Jonah said this prayer to the LORD, his God:

"Out of my distress I called to the LORD,
and he answered me.
From the midst of the nether world I cried for help,
and you heard my voice."
—*Jonah 2:1–3, New American Bible*

If the Lord heard Jonah crying out in prayer from within the belly of a large fish, think of how clearly he hears you as you pray to him in the hospital! This is a great comfort, indeed, when you, too, feel "swallowed" by the four walls of a hospital room and confined to a position of lowliness and infirmity. Instead of being cut off from your spiritual sustenance, you are still held up by the Lord, still protected by his steadying hand.

Of course, it must have been terrifying for Jonah to leave the open beauty of the world and slide down the fish's throat into utter darkness. So, too, it must have been frightening for you to go through the automatic doors of the hospital and put your life in the hands of innumerable strangers. From the orderlies to the nurses to the consulting physicians, you might never even be able to get to know these people by name, yet they are responsible for your health; because of their care, you will one day be able to go home.

Although there are artificial lights and perhaps glints of sun coming through the windows of your room, there is nevertheless a lot of darkness when you are in the hospital. You might have to be sedated because of pain, diagnostic procedures, or an operation, and this brings a physical "darkness" upon you that is difficult to see through. Also, many of the medical professionals attending you might be unable to answer your questions, and this could leave you "in the dark" regarding your progress or course of treatment.

In the hospital you are isolated from the outside world. You wonder how your household is functioning without you. You worry about your job, children, and plans that have to be altered or canceled. . . .

Truly, being confined to the hospital, like Jonah's experience in the belly of the fish, is a difficult place to have hope and faith. Surrounded by all of the activity and anonymity of the hospital, it is hard to find a quiet, meditative moment to pray. Yet, like Jonah, you can't give up!

Jonah did not have the luxury of a comfortable place or unlimited time in which to pray eloquently to the Lord. Rather, his supplication was simple and direct: "Out of my distress I called to the Lord, and he answered me." Taking your cue from Jonah, you don't have to wait until you are calm, cool, and collected: in your present state of distress and in unfamiliar and frightening surroundings, you can talk to the Lord . . . you *should* talk to the Lord, in whatever way you can. In this way your hope will be sustained and your faith will be strengthened, for you will know, deeply and surely, that you are never alone.

How long the days of Jonah's confinement must have been to him! Yet, he was in the belly of the fish only three days and three nights. As the days drag on for you in the hospital, you, too, might become despondent and impatient. But keep your prayer going and the days will fly by. Even if you cannot speak aloud because of tubes, medication, or your excruciating symptoms, the Lord can hear your tiniest whisper in the far reaches of your heart. And not only can he hear you—he will answer you and lead you back out of the darkness into the blessed light!

O Lord, I am so afraid of being in the hospital.
I do not like the darkness. I do not like my confinement.
But let me learn from Jonah's example and continue to
rely on your presence, protection, and Word.
That I might have hope and faith abundantly
from now until you lead me back into the light.

STARTING A NEW RELATIONSHIP

Do not be yoked with those who are different, with unbelievers.
For what partnership do righteousness and lawlessness have? Or
what fellowship does light have with darkness?
—*2 Corinthians 6:14, New American Bible*

There is a lot of thought that goes into starting a new relationship with someone after you have been diagnosed with a serious illness. Whether you are seeking a friendship or possibly a romantic tie with someone, you need to be sure that whomever you choose to let into your life will be able to understand, support, and nurture you compassionately, just as you will want to do in return. This knowledge isn't something that you can sense immediately upon meeting someone; it is gleaned through conversation and experience, through prayer and practice.

Making a new friend or spending time with someone you think might become your spouse is an important, exciting—and sometimes nerve-wracking experience. You ask yourself all sorts of questions.

"What if this person doesn't take my illness seriously?"

"What if I can't participate in the activities this person likes to do?"

"What if my illness gets worse and this person has to shoulder more of the responsibility in the relationship or marriage?"

"What if this person can't handle my illness and turns away from me?"

These questions might lead to serious doubt, even preventing you from pursuing a new relationship out of fear or lack of confidence. Or, if you do reach out to someone, you might find that there are fewer people equipped emotionally and spiritually to handle someone else's illness on top of all the other aspects of a relationship. Yes, you might be rejected—more than once—when you decide to reach out to people.

But this does not mean that you should give up. Rather, you should seek out new relationships among people who share your depth of spiritual discovery, who cling to prayer and listen, truly listen, to God's call in their lives. You should also look upon a new relationship as a two-way street; your illness should not be the center of it, but rather one aspect among many that make up the whole. In this way you will find common ground that goes beyond what you like to do on Saturday evening. You will find a basis for a more lasting communion and mutual compassion and respect.

In this reading from Corinthians, Paul urges his brothers and sisters to "not be yoked with those who are different, with unbelievers." Choosing to develop relationships with like-minded Christians is an excellent place to start your search for close friends and perhaps a soul mate. Although Christians are "people, too," and some might not be able to get past your illness, you will find among the fellowship of believers strong, faithful brothers and sisters in Christ—an excellent place to start. By widening your prayer circle and making friends with others who are striving to do God's will, you are more likely to strengthen your own faith and find God more readily in the faces and smiles of those around you. Also, you will learn to be a friend, as much as you are a friend, to love, as much as you are loved.

In our darkest moments, when we are in horrible pain or

feel terribly alone, it is natural for us to wish we had someone with us to see us through, hold us, tell us it will "be all right." The more we rely on the Lord, however, we will find that he is the One who is always with us, who gives us nonstop comfort.

A new relationship with a man or a woman adds a human element to God's care and love for us, but it also brings us into a position to let God work through us. In reaching out to our brothers and sisters in Christ, we are continuing the presence of the Lord in our lives and in their lives—and setting the foundation for new relationships that are built with immense faith and trust in the Lord.

O Lord, help me find fellow believers
with whom to nurture faith-centered relationships.
Let me be as understanding of them as they are of me,
and let me keep the honor, integrity, and holiness
of your brotherhood and sisterhood
in all ways and all days.

A Deeper Faith

Faith is the realization of what is hoped for and evidence of things not seen.

—*Hebrews 11:1, New American Bible*

So many people want to have "proof" of the Lord's might and power, or even of his existence. Some modern archeologists, scientists, psychologists, study the minutest detail of history or the present to find "evidence" that faith is justified, and others put up very convincing arguments that what cannot be proven "must not exist." Christians, too, comb through ancient texts or excavation sites, hoping to find the one "link" that will demonstrate that the descriptions in the Bible or the people named in Scripture actually happened or existed. In this way they believe that nonbelievers will be converted and that they themselves will have a deeper, more profound connection with the Lord.

But should we wait for that text or rock-hewn tomb to suddenly deepen our belief to an unshakable certainty? It is part of human curiosity and also part of God's gift to the world that such things can be discovered. But is there more to faith than concrete things, which weather with age and eventually vanish?

If we allow ourselves to be guided by this reading from Hebrews, we know that faith is a vibrant, living thing. Far from being something that is carved or written, it is the "realization of what is hoped for." This makes faith something that is constantly moving, growing, and connected to us individually in a very profound way.

Our very hopes are connected with our faith. God's movement in our lives and the way in which those hopes are realized directly influence our faith. We don't need to look to a faraway place for our faith, nor do we need to rely upon the discovery of a new archeological site for our faith to grow.

Faith is rooted in the Word of the Lord and in the salvation given to us through the gift of his Son Jesus Christ. It lives and breathes through the actions that God sustains in and through our own lives.

In the same way, our faith is "evidence of things not seen." Faith is something tied to that which is alive, vital, ever-growing. We *show* it out of our belief and experience of the way God has moved in our lives. We have faith because God is working in us and in the world of Christians around us. Others can't necessarily see that work; sometimes it is so subtle and personal that only we sense it. But the proof of that work is borne by our faith, and *that* is something everyone can see by the things that we do and say and the way we look, the joy on our faces.

The longer I live with chronic, serious illness, the more I pray for my faith to be deepened. With each triumph over pain and hardship, with each glorious "good" day, I experience the realization of what I have hoped for. I can't necessarily *show* others, especially nonbelievers, that this is happening. I can't turn their hearts by merely telling them that it is through faith that I have been brought through the wilderness. But I do keep witnessing . . . and praying that someday they, too, will find the Lord in the real way that I have.

I still know that I need to have *more* faith because even more challenges will undoubtedly befall me. But I keep praying for this, because I know that it will not come from a statue or a new translation of a word within a book of the Bible. My faith will not be swayed by scientists or others who tell me that it can't be "valid" because it cannot be "proven."

No, my faith will come from the Lord's working in me and through me. It will come from the practical reality of allowing God to inhabit my being and turn my life into a divine process rather than from anything tangible and fleeting. How true is the Lord in my life! How marvelous if everyone were to believe!

> *O Lord, deepen my faith.*
> *Let me believe more assuredly that you are*
> *moving and working*
> *through my life and in the lives of others.*
> *By witnessing to your work, let me bring your message*
> *to others*
> *and let their and my faith be based upon*
> *a soul-deep belief,*
> *the evidence that goes beyond any other.*

TAKING NOTHING FOR GRANTED

God saw all that he had made, and it was very good.
—Genesis 1:31, New International Version

The variety in God's creation is enormous and amazing! Sometimes I am in awe of the things that God has created. Other times I think he has a tremendous sense of humor! I find breathtaking beauty in the dew that glistens on early-morning blades of grass. I laugh out loud at the many ways a dog will try to get the attention of its "human." The color palette the Lord has worked from is nothing short of astounding. The balance of all things to make this one world is truly without compare.

It is, I think, this balance of all things living and inanimate that makes me appreciate the world the most. All the organs of my body work to sustain life. The sea is "layered" with large and small fishes, vast expanses and tiny hiding places. We move in and out of one another's lives, giving and taking support, encouragement, and fellowship. All of this shows a balance and a harmony that are borne of God's genius and his love for us. It is no wonder, then, that we cannot take any part of this life and this world for granted. Rather, we can use our time of illness to notice what we haven't noticed before, and appreciate more greatly the totality of what is within and without us.

Indeed, this time of prayer and quiet reflection is perfect for seeing God's creation with fresh eyes and for realizing that nothing is so small as to be taken for granted. Beginning with your body, have you noticed how precious all aspects of your outer self are? If you are balding, think of the gift of your skin. If you are marked with rashes, think of the creams and salves that are available to help alleviate them. Don't neglect the things that aren't problematic, too. How amazing it is that you can grow fingernails!

Now, reflect on the internal. Have you thought about how much of a miracle your inner self is? How all your organs work together? How perfectly they all fit within your skin?

Think of the room you are in. Air moves through it so you can breathe. The light is just right for you to read this book. There might be subtle noises in the room, or perhaps a ringing in your ears, but no sound is too loud for you to hear God's voice clearly as you listen.

In your life there are things to see anew, or perhaps for the first time, so that you can develop a deeper gratitude for them, too. The way you acquired this book, perhaps. The conversation you had with your doctor. The laugh you shared with your spouse. The minor "crisis" you solved for your children.

In spite of your disability, you are able to do much more than you might think. You can communicate. You can give witness and comfort to others. You can appreciate God's nature and world. You can *feel* the depth of emotion that only human beings are given. You can cry and laugh.

You can live, be fully involved in the world—and rejoice.

On this day, savor each breath, each step, each moment as if you'd never experienced them before. Thank the Lord for his many gifts, great and small. And tell others about your remarkable discoveries, that they, too, might see this world in a new and different way.

And never again take anything for granted.

Peace in the Storm

O Father, sometimes I become so tunnel-visioned
that I don't pay attention to the small things in this
world, let alone the great things.
Help me to open my eyes and take time
to appreciate all of your creation
and encourage others to do the same
and experience the same deep wonder and joy.

MANAGING ANGER

Get rid of all bitterness, rage and anger, brawling and slander, along
with every form of malice.

—*Ephesians 4:31, New International Version*

Gardeners carefully tend their lawns with a diligence that is
to be admired. They cut, prune, fertilize, and rake so that
the grass might have enough nutrients and space in which to
grow. But despite all of their careful labors, gardeners are constantly battling the scourge of any well-kept, healthy lawn:
weeds.

Weeds come in all shapes and sizes. Some have interesting
leaves, others have startling colors, still others have pretty
flowers. But no matter how attractive they might seem, weeds'
roots and stems can penetrate the soil and take hold with an
iron grip, choking out the tender grass and making the lawn
appear patchy and ill tended. At their worst, weeds can take
over a lawn and reduce it to ruin.

There are two ways that weeds can come to a lawn:
through external means via seeds borne on the breeze or carried on feet and in grass seed or topsoil mixes, and internally
through a network of roots that spread beneath the lawn's surface. To combat weeds, gardeners first identify what they are
and how they proliferate. They then might apply chemicals
and natural products to kill them, or they might pry the weeds

out of the ground, tossing them aside. In all cases, however, gardeners must constantly be on guard against them and take immediate action to prevent their encroachment. Sometimes the weeds are eradicated for good. Other times they grow back stronger, choking out more grass and making the gardener work extra hard to control them.

The benefits of a weed-free lawn greatly outweigh the effort it takes to keep it that way; a lawn devoid of weeds is a healthy, vibrant, luxurious carpet of lush grass. It is a beauty to behold and a source of happiness and satisfaction for every good, diligent gardener.

Managing anger is much like controlling the weed population in your lawn. Anger can "crop up" through your internal struggles, especially with your illness, or can be piqued by external frustrations or challenges. It is certainly a natural part of living and being human, but if anger is allowed to take root, to fester in your heart, it can create terrible damage to your well-being and your soul. It can take away the attractiveness of being a Christian and take you farther from a life of holiness and joy.

Just as a gardener does, to eradicate anger in your life you must first identify what kind of anger you feel and where it comes from. Saint Paul's list of the types of anger is a good place to start when trying to discern what kind you feel: Is it bitterness? Rage? Brawling/physical? Slanderous? Malicious?

Once you identify your anger, you can take steps to rid yourself of it. Perhaps you need to work on internal "triggers" or attitudes, or perhaps you need to address external, environmental effects or relationships with others. You might want to seek the help of a medical professional to work out your anger. You might also want to turn to extra prayer, relying on God's cleansing forgiveness to put your anger into perspective and at last eradicate it from your life.

The more I live with chronic illness, the less angry I have

become. Truly, having withstood the extreme ups and downs of pain and suffering, I tend to be more immune to acute rages and frustrations. But I still need to be vigilant, just like the good gardener, and catch the "weeds" of anger early, before they take root. I want the lawn of my soul to be healthy, vibrant, and thriving. To do that, I need to get rid of all forms of anger and concentrate on nurturing what is good.

Lord Jesus, you have given me a wonderful
garden of emotions with which to experience life.
Please bring me peace and calm,
and help me diligently rid my soul of anger
in all of its forms,
so that I may grow richly and righteously
in your most holy presence.

BEING REALISTIC

There are different kinds of spiritual gifts, but the same Spirit; there
are different forms of service, but the same Lord; there are different
workings but the same God who produces all of them in everyone.
To each individual the manifestation of the Spirit is given for some
benefit.

—1 Corinthians 12:4–7, New American Bible

W hen you are diagnosed with a serious illness, you might
have the sensation of having your wings clipped. Your
former activities, relationships, even your lifestyle might have
to change or be stopped altogether because of the health crisis
in which you find yourself. In those early days and weeks following diagnosis, it is natural to fight the new reality a little.
A bird that has its ability to fly curtailed still flaps its wings,
sometimes frantically, trying to fly even when it cannot. So,
too, you might try to push yourself to keep up with your pre-
illness schedule. You might not tell a lot of people about your
diagnosis and thus make them think that "everything's still
fine." In many ways, large and small, you might "flutter your
wings," hoping deep inside that your diagnosis was all a mistake and your life will go back to the way it was, even though
it will not.

The more there is a disconnect between the reality of your
health and your actions and thoughts, the more you will "flut-

ter your wings" and feel ill at ease, unsettled, not at peace. Your activities could start to bring you physical harm and your relationships might suffer from your futile efforts. The bird that still tries to fly might break a wing. You might injure your heart as well as your body.

The Lord wants so much more for you than to live in never-ending pain and frustration! Beneath all of your denial and efforts to work against your physical condition, God is working a different reality within you. He is opening the door for you to discover the true gifts of the Spirit that he has bestowed upon you.

This time in your life, however traumatic, is part of the process of revealing God's will for you, his new reality for your life. It is your golden opportunity to discover the unique qualities and the precious spiritual gifts that he brings only to you.

It is very easy to get caught up in a rhythm of life and think that it is the only one for you. As routines develop and time passes, the day-to-day might seem, if not perfect, at least suited for you. Your choice of livelihood and lifestyle might be so ingrained in you that you might not be able to imagine doing anything differently.

But in drawing you into a world of illness, the Lord is giving you an opportunity to feel more deeply, to experience things that no one else can. And he is calling you to turn away from what you thought was reality for yourself and embrace a new life and find a new manifestation of the Spirit that is much more suited to your situation than any other could be.

Breaking away from the "routine" is always frightening. Moving from being "healthy" to being "sick" is also terrifying. But there is benefit to it, which the Lord knows well. And he will reveal this to you in his good time, if you stop trying to go back to the way things were and move on to the way things really are.

Truly, deep within you, God has given you individual, specific gifts through his Holy Spirit. The more time you spend in prayer, asking for discernment to be able to recognize them, the closer you will come to being fully and realistically the kind of person that you are meant to be—and you will soar!

O Lord, make me obedient to you
and realistic about the gifts that you are bestowing
upon me.
Help me to find deep within
the manifestation of the Spirit
and dwell in my new reality with a joyful,
willing heart.

Having a Bad Day

I consider that our present sufferings are not worth comparing with the glory that will be revealed in us.

—Romans 8:18, New International Version

Some mornings, I wake up and I just know it's not going to be a good day. Usually I have no warning of this; I can't find "bad day" on my calendar and anticipate it the evening before. I can't "bad day–proof" my home or body, either. No matter the precautions I might take, bad days just seem to "happen," and when they do, I have to drop everything (which on a bad day can be both literal and figurative) and adapt.

This wasn't always the case. I used to fight through bad days. Pretend they weren't happening. "Push through" the pain or ignore all the "little things" that went wrong. But instead of making the day better or more pain-free, things just seemed to get more muddled. So now I accept bad days and try to take them in stride. And the reading from Romans certainly helps me do just that.

Reflecting on the perspective that Saint Paul gives us, I begin to open up my thoughts beyond expecting that heaven is the opposite of my world of illness and suffering. The "glory that will be revealed to us" is more than someplace devoid of pain, absent of glitches, and free from worry. It is something so much greater, so much better, that there *is* no comparison.

How marvelous is that?

Moreover, if I look at my limited experience with suffering, I find that it is nothing compared to what some other people go through, and certainly nothing in light of the suffering and death of our Lord Jesus Christ. Even when I amass all of the things that can go wrong in the "ultimate bad day," I cannot truly say that I am beset by misfortune. After all, what is a broken glass or missed appointment or bout of the flu compared to the suffering of starving children or the sense of betrayal Jesus must have felt at the hands of his human "friend" Judas?

In prayer and meditation, I've come to wonder recently if the days I've thought of as "bad" are truly that. Is any day when I awaken and have some semblance of a life a "bad" day? Is getting caught in traffic the equivalent of carrying a splintering cross on my back? Is all of my suffering worth "comparing with the glory that will be revealed to us"?

And if I have that incredible, awe-inspiring promise of salvation, how bad can anything be?

There's no denying that some days are more challenging than others. Some flares of an illness are worse, certainly, than remission. And sometimes, despite our best intentions, nothing we do seems to come out right. But in all of this, we still have hope.

The next day could very well be much better. The flare could subside quickly. New miracles and manifestations of our Lord can reveal themselves at any time, in any way. Even if we must endure a string of "bad days," our faith will grow from adversity and our strength will be refined.

And above and beyond all of this, we know profoundly, deep within our very souls, that the promise of the Resurrection is ours.

We cannot fully comprehend the magnitude of God's love for us. With our limited human senses, we cannot see, touch, or hear the whole of the glory God has in store for us. We *can* have faith and trust that all of our suffering, great and small, will pass away. And we will be able to praise our God for all eternity, free from pain, difficulty, or sorrow.

With this heavenly perspective, and with the example of Jesus upon our hearts, just how "bad" can a "bad day" really be?

O Lord, I know that you do not take my suffering
lightly.
But I know, too, that you have a heavenly reward
in store for me
that I cannot fully comprehend.
Please help me work through this "bad day"
with more hope and faith in you.
And please let me keep my eyes on the "prize" that you
will reveal to me,
and the glory that you have promised.

MARY'S "YES"

Mary said: "Behold, I am the handmaid of the Lord. May it be done
to me according to your word."
—*Luke 1:38, New American Bible*

Have you said "Yes" to your illness yet? Not a tacit acceptance or a grudging "Oh, all right."

A wholehearted, unequivocal "Yes!"

Long ago in Nazareth, a young woman was visited by an
angel of the Lord. He *told* her (he didn't ask her permission)
that she would give birth to a son and call him Jesus. It didn't
matter that Mary was a virgin. The angel assured her that she
would conceive of the Holy Spirit and her baby boy would be
the Son of God!

Mary's response to the angel has echoed through the centuries. Without doubting anything of what God intended to
do, she said, "Yes." And the whole world was transformed forever.

There is a deep sense of service in Mary's reply, and a great
humility. She saw herself not as someone exalted, but rather as
a "handmaid of the Lord." She wondered how God would accomplish what the angel told her; she was, after all, an intelli-
gent young woman. But she never questioned that she would
obey the Lord, even if it meant a world of problems and hurt
for her later on.

To get to this point of unwavering "yes" in our own lives is to achieve a depth of faith that takes time, prayer, and practice. It is easy to say "yes" to the good things, to a promotion, a child, a life of happiness. But to embrace *all* of God's will for us without doubt is difficult at best and a struggle of gigantic proportions when you have a serious illness.

For one thing, meaning "yes" takes away all ability to bargain out of pain and suffering. Fully accepting the Lord's will means you can't then say to him, "I'll accept this illness *if* you'll give it to me for just a few months" or "I'll accept this illness *if* you'll let me win the lottery." When we say we'll allow the Lord to work in our lives, we mean just that. Always. Everywhere. Every way.

Agreeing to the Lord's will for us also means we cannot go back on our word. In this we have the awesome example of Jesus, who did not waver as he walked the long road up to the hill where he was crucified. Once God's will is accepted, we, like Jesus, are on a divine path. Once we have let the Lord into our life, he will never forsake us.

Did Mary know what her "yes" would mean to her personally, and to the world? We don't have an answer to that in Scripture. But because Mary was a human being, we can imagine that she didn't fully grasp the full implications of her wholehearted agreement with what the angel told her would happen. Her faith, though deep and true, was probably a bit blind to what her response would mean to her life. And there is no mention in Scripture, either, that she had any hint of the suffering her dear Son would have on Calvary.

Saying "yes" to God is probably the most intimate, personal thing we will ever do. That one word invites the Lord to work in us divinely, completely. It does not guarantee that we will be free from suffering. But it does seal our relationship with the Lord and takes us on a blessed journey full of glory, light, and salvation.

Peace in the Storm

O Lord, let my "yes" to you ring as truly and
completely
as Mary's did so long ago.
Help me to embrace your will for my life
with all of my heart and energy.
And let me follow where you would lead,
no matter the place or time.

BEING A FRIEND

"You shall love your neighbor as yourself."
—*Mark 12:31, New American Bible*

You know the song "What a Friend We Have in Jesus." Well, I think we illness sufferers could sing another song, too: "What a Friend We Have in Each Other."

Friends are truly most precious to us when we have a chronic, serious illness. I know of no stranger who would listen so patiently as I go through my list of symptoms on any given day. I know of no medical professional who could "prescribe" the human anecdote to frustration and isolation like the presence of a good friend. In friends, we have sisters and brothers who will bear our foibles, understand our "bad days," and bring us humor, encouragement . . . and chicken soup.

How much I appreciate my friends!

Sometimes I feel like such a slug that it's hard to get on the phone and have a good old-fashioned "yak-fest." But the beauty of a good friendship is that my friend will understand me when I say, "I'm not at my best today," and not turn away! My friends have driven me to labs for long tests, held my hand when I've been too weak to move, brought me food and picked up my prescriptions, and kept me in their prayers through good and difficult times alike.

With my friends, my life has been sweeter, happier, more joyful.

Yes, I cannot imagine living without my friends! And I so want to be a good friend back.

We all know that friendship is not really an even give-and-take relationship. We cannot measure the amount of support we receive and give it back in exactly the same amount or manner. But it is important to remember that even at our lowest point, a friend will need us to be a friend back. And when we are stronger, that same friend will need us, too. Often, however, it is difficult to do this because of our own health issues. As much as I would like to be able to sit with a friend in the hospital, for instance, I know that because of the immuno-suppressive drugs I am on, if I were to do that I might subject myself to dangerous infection.

There have been times when I've been too sick to attend weddings, funerals, or other important events in my friends' lives. And sometimes I've been asleep when a friend has called me to talk over a problem.

It would be easy to become self-absorbed because of illness. It would be easy to take the love and support from my friends and not try to be a friend in return because of the "excuse" of being too sick. But that is hardly a Godlike attitude and does not nurture a friendly relationship, but rather eventually will wear it out.

As I've lived with the ups and downs of lupus, I've tried to find ways to be a friend, to love my neighbor, in spite of my illness. Through prayer and thought, I've discovered that there are many creative ways to extend friendship and support, and I'm still on the hunt for others.

Above all, I've come to understand that in letting friends know I am trying, in telling them how much I love them and want to be a friend, too, I am coming close to fulfilling what our Lord wishes us to do.

In striving to be a friend, I think we live one of Christ's most important exhortations for us: "You shall love your neighbor as yourself." Our Lord Jesus gave his very life for his "neighbors," his children. What an example that is for us, especially on the days when we can run the risk of being so very self-centered.

Taking care of our health is an act of love for self that is vital to our living a Christlike existence. Taking care of our friends, too, is Christlike in nature and just as important. We want the best for our lives and we want the best for our friends.

And we hold both in prayer, knowing that God wants what's best for all of his children, too.

> *O Lord, I love and cherish my friends.*
> *They are truly gifts sent from you.*
> *Help me to find ways to be a friend in return,*
> *and to be more Christlike in my life,*
> *in spite of and because of my illness.*

Facing Death

"For we know that if our earthly dwelling, a tent, should be destroyed, we have a building from God, a dwelling not made with hands, eternal in heaven."
—*2 Corinthians 5:1, New American Bible*

When you face a serious illness, you also face death squarely in the face. You might be young, middle-aged, older. You might be rich or poor, on the brink of starting a family or enjoying your grandchildren. It does not matter. Facing death goes along with serious illness, with the deterioration of your body and quality of life.

It is something you must do.

But it is not something that is pleasant or hopeful . . . until you realize that death leads to eternity with the Lord, to a heaven we cannot even imagine.

Being human, the first thing we probably do when we think of dying is all that we will leave behind. Loved ones. A business. Beautiful clothes. A pet.

We think, too, of all the things we enjoy that we will never do again. Travel. Fly. Snuggle. Sing.

By the time we finish thinking of all of our losses, we are probably very depressed. How can death be so glorious if we have to give up all of this "heaven on earth"? Oh, of course, we'll be leaving behind all kinds of unpleasant things, too. Taxes. Ill health. Traffic jams. Rude people.

But don't all of the benefits to living outweigh the negatives?

They do.

But they don't come close to the promise God has made to us, to the marvel of his Salvation and the gift of *his* heaven— an eternity with him!

Death is as natural a part of life as being born, loving, and working. And just like our lives and all that is in them, it is a gift from God, a stage through which we pass to get to be with him forever. As painful as the moments before it might be, in death there is no pain or suffering, no hurt or sorrow. Those who are left behind are on earth to mourn and remember. But those who pass through the portal of death are in heaven to praise God all the rest of their days and beyond.

It is a great comfort to know that when our bodies are tired and spent, we will pass through to a "building from God, a dwelling not made with hands." And although it is difficult to accept the suffering we will have to endure in this world, especially as we cope with illness, it is a great joy to know that heaven awaits us. Would that everyone felt this joy; for, sick or healthy, each day that passes brings each person closer to eternal life.

Our faith, the same faith that makes us strong and brings us closer to the Lord, will be the key to hope and welcome as we come closer to death. It will allow us to reflect on God's goodness and love, his mercy and might. It will also be an example for others who fear death even more than we do; seeing us face death bravely and readily will surely inspire others to do the same.

Just as it is necessary to prepare our earthly affairs for our ultimate passing, so too is it important for us to prepare our hearts and souls. We love many people in this world, and we enjoy many things in it.

But we are not *of* this place, after all. We are travelers belonging to God who have not yet arrived at our destination.

Finally, however, we will let go of this "earthly dwelling" and be with the Lord.

What a glorious day in eternity that will be!

O Lord, I am human and I am afraid of death.
Help me calm my soul and heart
and prepare my spirit for moving from this life
into the glorious eternity that you have promised,
into the heaven where I will dwell with you forever!

DID I DO SOMETHING WRONG?

He delivered us from the power of darkness and transferred us to
the kingdom of his beloved Son, in whom we have redemption, the
forgiveness of sins.

—*Colossians 1:13–14, New American Bible*

The blame game. It is played in all arenas of this world, in all professions and stages of life, even in the realm of serious illness.

People get cancer because they were smokers.

People get diabetes because they can't control their weight.

People get lupus because they don't know how to control stress.

People get hepatitis C because they lived immoral lives.

People get AIDS because they were sexually irresponsible.

The list of blame is almost endless. And underneath it is a kind of punishing animosity for those people who "brought illness upon themselves." Sometimes it might seem as though people who become ill because of some action on their part (or inaction) are worthless or deserve to be sick. Oh, there could be some validity to the connection between certain actions or practices and contracting an illness. But as harsh as this can be (and sometimes is), society's stigmas are often much more unforgiving.

What about you? Do you wonder if you did something to

bring about your illness? Do you *know* that you did? Does that change your perspective on your life and health? Do you feel worthless because of it? Or undeserving of sympathy or understanding?

How has your feeling about yourself and your actions affected your relationship with others? How has it affected your relationship with the Lord?

Have you given much thought to God's love for you? Do you believe in his redemption and forgiveness?

I know this seems like a lot of questions, but it is important to consider them. In order to benefit from your medical care and get on with your life in a positive way, you will need to move from guilt to forgiveness, from feeling "dirty" to feeling "cleansed."

The Lord wants to welcome you to him with open arms. He wants to pour his forgiveness over you and protect you from "the power of darkness."

He knows you. He knows what you have done.

But he also loves you completely and forever. There is nothing he cannot do for you, there is no obstacle in the way of his total mercy and comfort for you.

You are his child.

He is your Father.

Can you accept this?

No matter what you have done, the Lord will bring you into his light if you open yourself to him. If you fill your heart and soul with his Word and with the prayer of one who seeks, he will be there for you and lead you onward. Society's stigmas are nothing compared to the glory the Lord has in store for you as his precious creation, his beloved son or daughter. In him, there is no fear, no guilt. Only salvation.

But open your time to prayer and your heart to him, live according to his Word and guidance, and he will set you free.

I pray for you each day and night that you can do this. For

it is in God's forgiveness that we have the full power to become whole again, to "heal" in the fullest sense of the word, body and soul.

Gracious God, I know that I have erred.
Help me through my guilt into your light of forgiveness.
Let me live forevermore in the shadow of your
protective wings.
And let me move from darkness into light,
from the sense of worthlessness to the knowledge
that I am your precious child.

PATIENCE

I wait quietly before God
for my hope is in him.
—*Psalm 62:5, New Living Translation*

Hurry up . . . and wait.

That is the way it is so often in the healthcare field. You set an appointment to see a specialist and arrive early so you can fill out all the paperwork before your scheduled time. And you end up waiting for one, two, three hours anyway! Or your doctor says that you *must* have a special scan to know exactly what's happening inside your body, but you must wait weeks before there is an opening to "fit you in." Often, medication does not work overnight and you must wait for it to begin to work, "grinning and bearing it" in the meantime. Or a disease might not manifest itself completely all at once, and you and your doctor must wait, like vigilant "spies," until it appears in a blood test or a clinical examination in order to be able to proceed with treating it.

As patients, we have to have a lot of patience. And that is not easy when we are suffering and the minutes seem to stretch into eons. The outside world doesn't help, either; we live in such an instant society that people have come to expect instant results—hardly helpful when waiting for medication or insurance approval.

Over time, I'm sure each one of us has had someone ask, "Aren't you cured (or in remission) yet?"

Patience can be the most elusive of virtues in the middle of the night when your body is breaking down and you're waiting for the doctor on call to return your page. It can be completely nonexistent when all of the pressures of your illness combine with those of everyday life and make you utterly inconsolable. To be sure, it is something to strive for. But I have to admit, I fall short of it frequently.

I often count the very minutes during the time that I have to wait, and my impatience mounts with each sweep of the second hand. Or, if I am patient, I might still fill the time with all sorts of "busywork" in hopes that my activity will make the time pass that much faster, even though all that seems to do is sap me of energy later on.

How do we get to the ideal point of patience where we "wait quietly before God"? The key is, I believe, in the second part of the reading: ". . . for my hope is in him." This is not an inactive hope, but a fully engaged feeling of giving the Lord all of our worry and urgency and letting him move the mountains in our way. If we keep this in mind, then our energy will be spent lifting up problems in "idle" time and in doing so filling our moments with focus on him. Then our hearts will be quiet. We will be able to wait patiently, knowing that God is in charge of all else.

Acquiring patience, like any other virtue, takes time and practice. We won't succeed every time in not being frantic, snappish, or discouraged when we have to wait a long time for something. In truth, we need patience to be patient patients! But the more willing we are to let the Lord take over the time during which we wait, the more energy we will have for his glory and our health and well-being.

In being patient, we come to a greater understanding that God's time is not our time, but he *is* ours for all time. What a blessing to know that we can wait in the presence of God instead of with folded arms and tapping toes.

What a blessing to know that God controls the clock and we have only to "wait quietly" while his will unfolds.

O Lord, let me learn more patience
and practice it with joy,
recognizing that your time is not my time
and that you hold me up and protect me
even as I wait for your will to unfold.

PRESERVING YOUR DIGNITY

In you, LORD, I take refuge;
let me never be put to shame.
—*Psalm 71:1, New American Bible*

We have each suffered some form of indignity through our illnesses. Sometimes, in fact, the treatments are worse than the disease, at least in a temporary way. It is so very easy to lose sight of the grandeur of God's creation when we're writhing in pain, bleeding copiously, or heaving because of chemotherapy. Why, not too long ago we used to worry if there was food stuck in our front teeth. Now, some of us wonder if anyone will notice that we don't have any hair!

The physical effects of illness can rob us of our sense of dignity. So, too, can the other effects of illness. Finances, for example, can become so tight that a patient might miss payments on his or her car or house. The shame from such a lapse can become so heavy a burden that the same person who was very responsible prior to being ill might end up financially bankrupt.

For some, not being able to move freely is a shameful sign of weakness; they would rather not move from their homes if it means people seeing them using a cane or a walker. And people who experience speech difficulties following a stroke might feel very ashamed that they can't express themselves as freely as they once did, so they might not try speaking at all.

As we look over these many things that can bring "shame" upon a person who has a serious illness, we might think that all of them are really quite small when compared with the life-altering reality of a terrible sickness. Someone who loses their home because medical bills drain their money shouldn't be ashamed, should they? Someone who has to get by in a wheelchair shouldn't feel weakened, should they?

Actually, some people in our society would say that they should. Some people do perceive ill health, bad financial conditions, or other tangible misfortunes as evidence that a person is less than "worthy."

But in the eyes of God, we are all most worthy. We are all precious. So, too, in our eyes, we must be loving, putting no one to shame, including ourselves.

Taking refuge in the Lord, we turn away from shamefulness and toward our holiness in him. True, it is not glamorous to go through chemotherapy, but in God's eyes we are still his beloved children no matter how badly we react to the treatment.

Knowing that God will provide for us whatever we require if our finances become terrible, we need not be ashamed, but keep our hope and trust in him.

Facing our infirmity, we pray for strength, and God will see us through and give us courage.

As we pray "Let me never be put to shame," we take off embarrassment and put on the robe of goodness that God gives us. We learn to laugh with our individuality, our "quirks" that make us uniquely ourselves. And we learn to handle the negative remarks of others, who have not achieved the same kind of depth of faith and charity that we have. At least, not yet.

Being confronted by others who think we are shameful is a good opportunity to instruct them, gently and calmly, on God's love for each of us and his acceptance of who we are. It is an excellent chance to tell them that no matter what trouble befalls us, we are still precious in God's eyes, still heirs to the Kingdom.

The lack of hair on your head, the limp in your step, the retching, the financial struggle are no more "shameful" than having a piece of food stuck in your teeth. Truly. The Lord will preserve your dignity through all this and more. You will never be put to shame if you take your refuge in him.

O Lord, in my illness I see myself as so undignified.
But I know that you see me as your child,
full of faults, but lovable even so.
Please bring me to you, let me take my refuge in you.
And let me find dignity where others would bring me
shame,
and righteousness where I would be afraid.

Nurturing Your Dreams

Search me, O God, and know my heart;
test me and know my thoughts.
Point out anything in me that offends you and lead me along the path of
everlasting life.
—*Psalm 139:23–24, New Living Translation*

Think back to the days when you'd watch the clouds waft by in all their myriad shapes and spin dreams in your mind and heart. What did you most want to do or be "when you grew up"? Was it to be a firefighter? To join the circus? To climb a mountain? To be a mother?

Now that you have a serious illness, you probably think those dreams are so far removed from your reality that they are no more valid than the well-worn teddy bear you used to play with but that now sits neglected on a shelf in the back of your closet.

It is true that there might not seem to be much in common between what you dreamt as a child and what you are living through now. You've been through so very much lately that the more innocent dreams of your youth probably seem like filmy cotton candy now that you are forced to eat bitter licorice. But this time, now when you are suffering from illness, is exactly the right time for you to dust off those childhood dreams and nurture them and perhaps others.

For there is nothing like a chronic, serious illness to make us realize that time is precious, that this life is special, and that we should, in all things good, make the most of it that we can.

This is not to say that we should throw aside all of our responsibilities. But with our adult ability to plan and our Christian faith in God's power—and with a healthy dose of childlike wonder—we need to spend time dreaming . . . and seeing some of those dreams through to fruition.

Our dreams need not be grandiose or elaborate. They can be as simple as going for a trail ride, traveling to a place we've always admired, or finally learning to play the flute. They could be tied to our relationships with others; maybe there is someone in your family you've always dreamt of spending more time with. Now is that time.

Perhaps our dreams are not attainable in exactly the way we'd originally thought; you might not be able to join the fire-fighting brigade in your hometown. But you could volunteer one weekend to cook for the squad or help in some other way.

Have you always dreamt of writing a book? You have only to take pen to paper to get started. One page a day, and you'll have a complete volume in less than a year!

Are you having trouble remembering what it was that you dreamt about as a child? In spending quiet and close time in prayer, God will search your heart and reveal to you things that you've probably forgotten but, once revisited, can rekindle your excitement and energy in a very vibrant way. You will not just be going back to former dreams, you will be creating a new reality for yourself that will bring a new, alive feeling to your present condition.

Without dreams, our suffering seems dire indeed and often devoid of hope. But with dreams, with something to look forward to, we are brought out of our suffering in a wonderful way. We learn to challenge ourselves to *live* and exercise the many gifts that God has given us.

By dreaming, we are lifted out of the mundane and brought closer to our Lord.

Nurturing dreams is an important part of maintaining your health in body, mind, and spirit. It is, of course, important to be realistic. But it is also important to go beyond the confines of your current life and routine and discover the new/old aspects of who you are as a creation of the Lord and a very vital human being.

The next time you see clouds up in the sky, in all their many forms, remember your dreams. And as the clouds drift by, begin to think of ways to make those dreams come true.

With God's help and your imagination, anything is possible!

O Lord, let me be childlike in my wonder and
my dreaming.
Help me to find hope in my innermost thoughts
and prayers.
Bring me to a place where I can freely imagine
and then find a way to make my dreams
come true.

Overcoming Obstacles

Then Jesus looked at them and said, "For human beings, it is impossible, but not for God. All things are possible for God."
—*Mark 10:27, New American Bible*

We have all heard this phrase so many times that it might have lost the "edge" to its meaning. When we have faced challenges or been with others who have, the phrase "nothing is impossible for God" comes quickly to mind and is spoken often. Our response to it, "Yes, I know," is quickly spoken, too.

But how much of this revelation have we truly taken to heart?

There is nothing more daunting than facing a serious illness. It isn't like cramming for a test and it isn't like making a life-altering decision. When a sickness invades your life, you must gather all of your resources, internal and external, and arm yourself for a fierce, long-term battle. Throughout it there will be obstacles to seeing clearly beyond the suffering, to surviving. And, although you *know* that with God all things are possible, in the day-to-day humanness of the fight, the depth of your faith in this truth can be less than secure. As you parry and thrust your way through a jungle of problems, you might become filled with skepticism that God himself would be able to solve all of them. Or you might think that he is picking and choosing, electing to help you with some troubles and leaving others solely to you.

God understands your doubt and knows your fears. He acknowledges your humanness and recognizes that you cannot handle *everything* yourself. He intervenes on many occasions, sometimes in ways that you can't immediately see. And he moves mountains for you, even if it is inch by inch so that you can have relief.

If we were alone, away from the Lord, we'd be lost almost the moment we stepped into the jungle. We wouldn't have hope, we wouldn't have faith in God or even in ourselves. But with the Lord, our lives are completely transformed. Besides solving our problems, God works the impossible within us, removing some of our humanity and replacing it with the divine. He moves us to see his glory, feel his strength, and witness to his might. He calls us his children and pours his love upon us through all of our pain and sorrow.

Sometimes God lets us have our obstacles so that we can see just how marvelously he moves them through our efforts. He's not being mean to us, and he's not being sadistic. He's being a gentle parent, a loving teacher. The One who created each of us wants us to be as strong and resilient as we possibly can be so that others might know just how awesome faith in God is. Through our trials he makes us better people, people of light and hope—people that the world *needs* to see more of.

When everything is going along well, we sometimes forget to pray. In our human way, we dance along quite happily until we come up against an obstacle—*then* we pray! But truly, if we didn't have troubles to battle and problems to solve, we would never be able to do God's remarkable work or feel his all-encompassing love for us.

Doesn't this change the whole meaning of the word "obstacles" from something dreadfully negative to something positive? Doesn't it give a deeper meaning to the Scripture reading from Mark?

Overcoming obstacles is a huge part of the Christian experience, and it is something God wants us to do, something that we should welcome. Not that we *look* for trouble, illness, or other problems. But when they occur, we should look upon them as gifts that will only make us better Christians. We should invite the Lord into our troubles and open ourselves to letting him work through them, no matter how much we fear them. For God, nothing is impossible. And we should never forget to praise him every day for bringing us through the jungle!

> *O Father in Heaven, be by my side as I face*
> *the many obstacles*
> *that come my way each day and night.*
> *In my humanness,*
> *bless me with your strength,*
> *and in my weakness,*
> *let me reach a new depth of faith and hope*
> *with each battle that is won,*
> *and each obstacle that is overcome with you.*

WHEN THE TESTS BRING PAIN

Thus the LORD blessed the latter days
of Job more than his earlier ones.
—*Job 42:12, New American Bible*

You wouldn't think that diagnostic tests could bring more pain than the actual illness, but sometimes they do. Even a tiny skin biopsy or needle prick can cause scars, bruises, rashes, or other disfigurement. Lying on an X-ray table can cause cramps, back spasms, and chills (those tables are always so very cold!). Having tubes snaked down the esophagus or through the intestines can bring soreness for days.

The aftermath of tests can also be difficult to handle, filled with exhaustion, discomfort, frustration, and anxiety about what the results will be. Seldom do the lab technicians give indications of how things have gone, so we have to wait until a report is generated, read, evaluated, and sent to our attending physician.

And if the test has gone awry and you have to do it all over again?

I've seen many unhappy women get called back to the lab for additional mammograms because the first ones didn't come out very clearly; I can't blame them for complaining about it.

Early in my walk with lupus, I realized that I would have to undergo many different tests. To try to make taking them more palatable, I have sat with friends and played "Go Fish" and "Old Maid." I have put on headphones and listened to soothing Hawaiian music. I have worked crosswords, acrostics, word searches, anagrams, and all kinds of other puzzles. I have befriended the lab technicians and learned all about their families and foibles. In my mind, I have focused on a balmy summer evening by the ocean or an afternoon sitting in my favorite chair, reading. And, of course, through all of this, I have prayed.

But some tests still bring pain, and no matter how hard I try, I cannot escape it. When it does come, I try to separate my feelings of frustration and anger from the discomfort of the procedure and my disease. Breaking down my emotions like this enables me to manage what's happening in "small pieces" instead of one ugly "whole."

I try to remind myself that the pain from undergoing a test is usually short-lived. Also, thankfully, many diagnostic procedures have to be done only once (provided they are performed correctly the first time). It is with this thought that I take to heart this reading from Job: "Thus the Lord blessed the latter days of Job more than his earlier ones." Having come through the fire of some truly awful tests, I know now that my suffering from them was temporary, and the results, however negative, will be helpful in determining what course of treatment is necessary. Reflecting on this in the midst of horrible test moments helps.

Really, it does!

True to his Word, once again the Lord brings something good out of something unpleasant. He takes us through our discomfort and brings us safely to the other side of it.

After a harrowing experience in the hospital labs or doctor's office, take time to be good to yourself. You *have* been through an ordeal. Also, praise the Lord for being with you through thick and thin, and for allowing you to leave the pain behind and move on. For he blesses "the latter days" more than our "earlier ones."

Think of it.

From here onward, it will just keep getting better and better.

Really, it will!

O Lord, be by my side when I have to undergo tests
that frighten me, hurt me, or make me angry.
Help me to keep close to my heart that living in your
Promise
means that my future days will be more blessed than
the ones before,
and that my pain is fleeting,
but your love is abiding.

THE PROMISE OF LAZARUS

Jesus told [Martha], "I am the resurrection and the life; whoever
believes in me, even if he dies, will live, and everyone who lives and
believes in me will never die. Do you believe this?"
—*John 11:25–26, New American Bible*

On the surface of it, Jesus' words to Martha are confusing.
On the one hand, the Lord is saying that whoever believes in him, *even if he dies*, will live. But on the other hand,
he says that everyone who lives and believes in him "will
never die."

So, which is it?

Do we live, or do we die?

Amazingly, we do both!

Just as Jesus was the ultimate friend to Lazarus, so too is he
our ultimate friend. He gives us life here on earth and he gives
us life with him in heaven.

Our bodies will eventually die (stop living) on earth, but
our souls will never die.

The story of Lazarus is such a study in faith, miracle, and
substance that I can never read it and be bored. Rather, I am
inspired by the love Jesus had for his friend and the way he
carried out his miracle of raising Lazarus from the dead.

I'm also heartened by the women of the story: Martha,
who scolded Jesus for not coming sooner, before Lazarus died,

and Mary, who sat at home while Martha went out to meet the Lord. These two women are so human that they make Jesus' miracle of raising Lazarus from the dead all the more amazing. Aren't they just like some people we know?

Aren't they just like we are sometimes?

Not only do I revel in the resurrection aspects of Jesus' miracle upon Lazarus, but I also see another relevance to my life with illness:

No matter how ill I am, even unto death, my soul and my connection with the Lord continue.

I could be unconscious, and God would still be with me.

I could be so ill that I can't even carry on a coherent conversation, and the Lord will maintain a living, breathing dialogue with me, all the while holding me up lest I fall.

The Lord's nearness is so palpable that I can see him all around me and hear his voice inside no matter how deaf or blind I might be.

His glory reveals itself to my innermost core, and he makes sure that, when I need him most, he extends his healing hand so that I may rise from whatever tomb I am in and walk out into the daylight.

I've always wondered at how Lazarus felt, being dead one moment and raised to life the next. Was he stunned? Grateful? Confused? Did his eyes hurt from the sun? Did his bones feel stiff and his muscles cramped?

I can only imagine the thoughts and emotions going through Lazarus' head as he looked around and saw his beloved sisters, other neighbors, and Jesus at the mouth of his tomb. I have to believe, though, that he probably looked behind him, into the dark abyss and at the massive stone that had been rolled aside from it, and shook his head in wonder that he had made it out at all.

And I am sure that one look at his friend Jesus probably told him everything.

Although I might not be able to consciously feel the Lord with me at all times, I do know he is there. And after a dark moment, I sometimes look back to see how far God has brought me. There have been many dark tombs, but so, too, has there been salvation, with my friend Jesus standing right nearby.

I am always stunned and so very, very grateful that the promise of Lazarus is *my* promise, too, on this earth and in heaven above.

> *Father, I believe what you say,*
> *that you are the resurrection and the life.*
> *I know you are near at all times, and I know that you*
> *raise me up*
> *just when I would fall.*
> *Help me to appreciate all that you are to me,*
> *and let me have faith in our friendship,*
> *which guides and sustains me.*

Going through
Rehabilitation for
Addiction to Prescription
Medication

Because we have these promises, dear friends, let us cleanse our-selves from everything that can defile our body or spirit. And let us work toward complete purity because we fear God.
—2 Corinthians 7:1, New Living Translation

You have acknowledged that you are addicted to prescrip-tion medication. This realization brings to you a new re-solve: you will beat the addiction. So you enter a treatment program, fully prepared for it to be difficult but expecting that the results will far outweigh the struggle.

But your resolve flags quickly.

You didn't expect it to be *this* hard.

You didn't expect it to be *this* painful.

You didn't expect it to take *this* much time.

And you didn't expect life after rehab to be so troublesome.

For even after your body has been cleansed of the addictive substances, you have to fight your human impulses to regress, to go back to your addictive behavior. Indeed, you might fall back and end up in rehab again and again.

Addiction might become a cycle that seems impossible to break.

The harsh truth is that there is no drug that will give you the willpower and resolve you have to maintain to keep clean after being addicted to anything, especially prescription drugs. In many ways your struggle to become *un*addicted might stay with you for the rest of your days. As you add this challenge to the other ones in your life, you might become discouraged and depressed.

How do you get through this day-to-day battle?

How do you stay true to your initial resolve and the Lord's hope and expectation for you?

Isn't it easier to just give in to addiction and not fight this terrible fight?

Just as you would celebrate your successes with others, it is vitally important to turn to others for strength and support at the times when your hope flags and your resolve weakens. In fact, many former addicts maintain contact with their mentors, "partners," and others instrumental in their initial treatment for addiction. Through shared struggle and suffering they can uphold one another's resolve and make the long, arduous days seem brighter and more hopeful.

Your doctor and other members of your medical team are also wonderful resources for you both during and after rehab. They can help you put your medical condition, illness, and pain into perspective and offer ways for you to continue to battle your addictive behavior and take charge of more aspects of your life.

Along with the realization that you need support from others, in rehab and in health, you must realize that just as your addiction did not take place overnight, so too will your rehabilitation not magically set you back on the right track for ever and for good. You will be engaged in a constant struggle, and sometimes this challenge will be much greater than you expected.

Do not be afraid to cultivate colleagues and friends in bad times as well as good. Be ready to uphold them, too, in their quest for purity. And pray together, as always, for strength and insight.

Be heartened! Be strong! Be well!

Heavenly Father, I so want to serve you from now on.
Give me strength, discernment, and courage
to cleanse my body
and fill my life with all that is good, holy, and pure.
So that I may enjoy your presence in all things
and people
all the seasons of my life.

BEING A WITNESS

"No one who lights a lamp hides it away or places it [under a bushel basket], but on a lampstand so that those who enter might see the light."

—*Luke 11:33, New American Bible*

There is a light within you that burns so brightly it illuminates the darkest moments and corners of your life. It warms you on cold days. It sustains you when your strength is low and you experience a kind of spiritual "power failure."

This light is your unique reflection of the Lord's creation and his work within you.

It is in your smile, your dance, your song.

It is in the way that you nurture yourself, the way that you pray, and the way that you praise God.

Yes, this light is wonderful and beautiful. But if you keep it all to yourself, if you "hide it away or place it under a bushel," it will likely burn whatever is holding it in or suffocate from lack of air.

Your soul will not thrive if all of God's creation and love is trapped inside you, away from others who desperately need its warmth.

But how do you take your light to others if you feel wretchedly ill?

How do you let others experience your joy with the Lord,

or other aspects of his manifestation in your life, if you cannot leave your room?

Your light, your wondrous spirit and reflection of God's awesome power, will go as far as you are able to go and shine wherever you place it. If you cannot go beyond your home, your light will manifest itself in the way you treat others when they visit or call you. If you are confined to the hospital, your light will burn for the many strangers and loved ones who attend you.

Your light is visible in the words that you write in e-mails, in letters. It is a brilliant blaze to others who live in darkness next door to you or across the street. Your voice carries your light when you receive telephone calls from telemarketers (yes, really!) and it wraps around the tired arms of the water delivery person who serves you.

The more fuel you give your flame through prayer and reflection on God and his Word, and the more oxygen you give it through "airing it" before others, the stronger it will burn and the more light it will bring to you and other people. Your spirit and soul thrive on regular witness and praise of God's creation. And when you bring your light in contact with that of others— what a bonfire of witness there can be! Indeed, when two forest fires merge, the effect is almost unstoppable. And when two or more Christians converge and blend their flames of witness, that power is truly amazing!

In the time when Luke wrote his gospel, there was no electric power, no fluorescent lighting. The flame from a lamp generated heat as well as light. People who came near it saw it and *felt* it; the closer they came, the more they were warmed by it. So, too, it happens with the flame of your spirit. You need not worry about flinging it far across the country; it will be most effective when you put it on a lampstand near you and let it gleam from your inner faith. People who come near will see this light, and they will also feel its warmth. Believers will understand and be inspired, and those who do not yet believe might very well be transformed.

So do not hide away your light. Let it shine all around you, illuminating your life and the way God works in it. Let it join the lights of others so that together they may grow even more powerful.

Give your light a lot of fuel and air and feel it sustain you through your pain and joy.

Be a witness and let your light help you see just how remarkable the presence of God can be.

O Lord, help me tend the light within me
so that I may pass it on
to everyone with whom I come into contact.
Help me bring your witness and truth to everyone, too,
and join others in building your marvelous kingdom
on earth.

CHANGING EATING HABITS

Better a dry crust with peace
than a house full of feasting with strife.
—*Proverbs 17:1, New American Bible*

When I was put on a high dose of prednisone for a long period of time, one of my doctors warned me about the possibility of gaining weight.

"Before you get that prescription filled," she said, "go into your kitchen and throw out everything that has salt, sugar, or fat in it."

Needless to say, my cupboards and refrigerator were very barren when I finished! But I was soon very thankful for the warning—my appetite was almost insatiable when I started taking that medication. If I hadn't rid my household of all those goodies, I would have quickly become many sizes bigger!

During those prednisone days, I struggled with completely changing my eating habits. No longer could I snack on candy or cookies, no longer could I indulge in pizza and other "fattening" foods. All the while that my body was crying out for "treats," I steeled myself against that call and *really* worked to change the years-old way of eating that I had previously enjoyed. I learned new recipes, forced myself to develop new tastes for exotic fresh fruits and vegetables. I "lived vicariously" through others who could eat things I could not (smelling chocolate, I learned, is not exactly eating it, but it isn't fattening, either). And I prayed constantly for fortitude and visualized a slim, trim me despite all the prednisone I had to take.

I will not say those days were easy. Rather, they were excruciatingly difficult. But I am eternally grateful to that doctor who warned me about prednisone; because I took those early precautions, I was able to keep my weight gain and bloat to a minimum. And, more important, I learned to enjoy more healthful eating, a habit I continue to this day.

The other thing that happened when I changed my eating habits was that I stopped thinking of food as something that "was" and began considering it for what it "does." That is, I learned to appreciate, even crave, foods that could provide me with more long-lasting good effects than those that, say, gave me a sugar rush but left me exhausted later.

The reading from Proverbs is, I think, significant as you work to change eating habits that have been with you since perhaps childhood. Too often we think of denying ourselves "goodies" as a kind of deprivation, and no one likes to be deprived. But if we think of adopting better eating habits as a positive thing, as "better" than the alternative, we will be able to change our attitude completely.

The food we eat is fuel for every one of our internal organs and our external ability to get around in the world. The more healthful food we eat, and the more diligent we are about fueling our bodies with good sustenance, the better we will feel and the stronger we will be to withstand the challenges of living with our illnesses.

If you were a country besieged by invaders, wouldn't you want the most awesome weapons to repel them? It's the same with the food you eat—good fuel makes for good function.

The pleasure of feasting on unhealthful food is quickly

turned into "strife" in the form of weight gain, sluggishness, and lack of nutritional balance.

The peace of mind that accompanies good eating habits cannot be understated, nor can the physical and spiritual benefits be ignored. God so wants us to do all that is good for ourselves and his glory.

With this positive inspiration and in changing our eating habits, we are not just nourishing our bodies, we are nourishing our souls.

Lord Jesus, I ask for strength
that I may put into my body food that is good for it,
food that will nourish and strengthen it.
Help me to make better choices about what I eat,
and let me not fall into temptation, but do all that
is right,
that I might find peace and leave behind strife.

PULLED FROM THE
BRINK OF DEATH

The living, the living give you thanks,
as I do today.
—*Isaiah 38:19, New American Bible*

What an amazing sight it is to behold a family who has just been informed that their loved one has been pulled from the brink of death! Tears of sorrow are transformed into tears of joy, and wailing is replaced by laughter. Praise upon praise to God sings from the mouths of these happy people. Gratitude toward all the doctors, nurses, and other medical professionals who attended their loved one is poured forth from them, too.

And what does the patient feel, having been saved from death?

There are stories of people who have had near-death experiences. Many describe being pulled toward a bright light and feeling a sense of well-being. Some talk of being reunited with long dead relatives or friends. Others even talk about not wanting to be sent back to the living.

If you have been pulled from the brink of death, you might be very grateful, but you might also not share the joyful abandon that your loved ones feel. It might take you time to come to terms with what has happened to you and what impact it will have upon the life you lead from now on. For, as Christians, we look forward to an eternal place with our Lord after we have died. If you have caught a glimpse of heaven, it is natural that you should have mixed feelings about being brought back to live here on earth a while longer.

As you sort through your feelings and thoughts about being given a kind of "second chance" at living, reflect upon the many blessings you have in this life. The joy of your loved ones is the most present and obvious; they are so very happy to have you with them! There is happiness, too, in having gone through the very darkest of moments and feeling God's hand pulling you along, saving you, as only he can.

Indeed, what you remember of your experience on the edge of death is another blessing. You have gone through what few have, and your witness to God's salvation and presence can be a great inspiration to others.

You might feel a deep sense of renewal as your spiritual eyes refocus on your present life on earth. Perhaps you believe you have been brought back for a purpose other than what you thought you had before your experience. Perhaps, too, you are filled with a longing to change aspects of your life that seem out of step with who you have become. Truly, awareness of the power of God will take a new and prominent place in your thoughts and heart as you reflect upon what you have been through and where you are now.

Although your loved ones are immediately praiseful, it might be a long time before you are fully comfortable with what happened to you. Explaining what you have gone through might seem impossible at first, but as you go along you will find better and more descriptive words to convey your brush with death.

Your near-death experience will become one of the many miracles in your life. Step by step, you will move along, bearing witness to these and other amazing works that only the Lord can do.

As a vital, very real part of the community of believers on earth, you will join the living and, like them, give thanks and praise and honor to him for all that he has done for you and all that he will reveal.

> *O Lord, I did not know at first how to react to being*
> *pulled from the brink of death.*
> *But I am confident that in this, as in all things,*
> *you will do only what is right and good for me.*
> *And so I give you thanks for my life.*
> *And I give you the praise for having control*
> *over every aspect of it.*

PEACE IN THE STORM

Jesus woke up, rebuked the wind, and said to the sea, "Quiet! Be still!" The wind ceased and there was great calm.
—Mark 4:39, New American Bible

In the eye of the hurricane. In the middle of a tornado. In the aftermath of a great earthquake and before the aftershocks . . .

There is peace.

While all around the winds might blow and the earth tremble . . .

There is peace.

In the storms in our lives, in the middle of the darkest hour . . .

There is peace . . .

Because God ordains it.

The Lord can command the winds and the water, the earth and the sky. With the simplest of words, he can say, "Quiet! Be still!" and it will be done.

In our hearts, too, we can experience a profound, strong peace at a word from the Lord.

We have to listen for it, we have to be watchful. We have to *believe* there is peace.

And we shall find it.

No amount of outside tempest can shake our calm when the Lord is in control of our craft. The floods will not overwhelm us, the winds will not blow us off course. Even in our fright and despair, God will not see us destroyed. We are precious to him. We are his children. We are beloved. And in all of this knowledge . . .

There is peace.

Our hands might slip. Our legs become useless. Our voice, sight, hearing might fail. Our health might fall apart. But if we hear those simple words from our Savior . . .

There is peace.

Everyone around us might criticize us, throw obstacles in our way, deny that we are even ill. But if we hold fast to God's presence within us and our lives . . .

There is peace.

Have you ever stood up in a boat in the middle of a lake? If you have, you know how dangerous that can be. When the apostles were out in the water and the storm came up, threatening their lives, the Lord stood in the midst of it all. If the apostles had forced him to sit down and be quiet, the miracle might not have happened.

But instead, the apostles, despite their terror, watched as Jesus defied the storm and commanded it: "Quiet! Be still!"

And it was.

In allowing Jesus to work, the apostles were witness to a great miracle.

So, too, by opening our hearts and souls to the Lord, even in our direst hour, we invite Jesus to work. And he will. He will speak simply and profoundly.

"Quiet!"

"Be still!"

And there will be peace.

Peace in the storm.

PEACE IN THE STORM

O Lord, in the midst of all my storms,
let me hear and feel your peace.
Let your calm and comfort pour over me like the most
precious balm.
And let me not be afraid of anything,
but know that you are in complete control.

FINDING IT HARD TO BE MOTIVATED

If you remain indifferent in time of adversity,
your strength will depart from you.
—Proverbs 24:10, New American Bible

"Use it or lose it."

This is the motto of many companies when it comes to vacation policies.

It is also the underlying principle of being able to maintain range of motion in our bodies, hearts, and souls.

If we don't use our muscles, they will atrophy and it will be harder and harder to get them toned again.

If we don't allow ourselves to feel deep, human emotions, we will become dulled to the joys of living.

And if we don't use the spiritual gifts we're given, we will surely lose them, too.

There will be times when we can't be active at all, times when our illness will prevent us from activity, thought, or talking. This isn't the same as the "indifference" mentioned in the above reading from Proverbs. It is a fact of life with serious illness.

What Proverbs is talking about is not caring about the gifts God has given us, about ignoring them or turning them away.

This is the peril we need to avoid, for if we turn away from what God gives us, we are denying him the opportunity to work through us. We are hiding our lamp under a bushel. We are not being true to our Christian faith.

And our ability to overcome trial and persevere will slowly leave us.

We need all the strength and courage we can get. So it is vitally important that we keep our motivation high when we face the challenges in our lives. If we say, "There's no way I can do this" or "I don't want to deal with this" when we face a problem, we run the risk of not having the strength to carry on, to get through our problems, to feel God's miracles.

Sometimes problems can multiply so quickly that we feel we don't have time to rise above each one before the next one looms large upon us. So we need to constantly give ourselves "spiritual pep talks," reminding ourselves of how we *can* make it through trials and keeping God's promises foremost in our hearts and minds. This can be very difficult, especially if we are in pain. From the depths of physical infirmity, it is quite a challenge to reach up to the heavens.

Scripture is a powerful tool, keeping us focused on God and speaking words for us when we don't have the health to do it ourselves. Asking loved ones to pray with us and for us is another wonderful way to overcome personal hardship and enlist the support of others when we most need it. Listening to inspirational music, reflecting on past triumphs, rereading a prayer journal that chronicles the many ways God has worked in the past—these are all marvelous ways, too, of finding motivation when it eludes us.

You will no doubt discover other ways to find and keep spiritual motivation as you continue your walk with your particular illness. *What* you do is not as important as *that* you do it and *how* you do it.

If we are lethargic in our spirit and "just don't care," the door to temptation and other evils will be wide open, inviting trouble instead of godliness. But if we *want* to have victory, we will find a way to do it. If we *desire* holiness, God will guide us to it.

"Use it or lose it?" That applies to our lives, certainly. But perhaps more important, when it comes to deciding to be motivated in the spirit, we should remind ourselves to "Choose it and use it."

> *O Lord, it is difficult for me*
> *to keep my praise going throughout my illness.*
> *It is also hard to keep motivated in other ways.*
> *Work within me and through my loved ones*
> *to keep the fire of spirit burning within,*
> *even on my worst days.*
> *And let my strength increase abundantly.*

COPING WITH THE DEATH
OF A LOVED ONE

No longer shall your sun go down,
or your moon withdraw.
For the LORD will be your light forever,
and the days of your mourning shall be at an end.
—*Isaiah 60:20, New American Bible*

About a year after I was diagnosed with lupus, and while in the midst of a terrible flare, my young brother died suddenly and inexplicably. I had just spoken with him two days before. There was an e-mail from him on my computer, which I hadn't even read yet. But without warning, he was suddenly silent; I couldn't even say "good-bye."

Because lupus can be a fatal illness, I had been dealing with my own mortality ever since my diagnosis. Coping with my brother's death was something else. He was my only sibling. He was my friend, my "partner in childhood crime." I would have expected that I should have died first, given my precarious health.

But he was gone.

The darkness that fell over me those days immediately following my brother's death was all-encompassing. He had passed away on the other side of the country. I never saw his body. I wasn't even sure what the circumstances were surrounding his death. I tried to piece the story together, but not even the e-mail, which I finally had the courage to open, yielded any clues. My mind ached from the effort of trying to *know*, and my heart ached with trying to *feel* what and why this had happened.

But still there was darkness.

I kept up an almost nonstop dialogue with the Lord during those dark days. I know that, had I not, I would have sunk even lower. In my pain, I felt him keeping me going, walking through the things I needed to do to plan my trip to the memorial service and the things I needed to say to friends and family. He also kept his hand upon my lupus and gently prodded me to keep taking my medication, work with my doctor, and do everything possible to rely on others to help me through. Gradually, with this constant communication with the Lord, I found light again and peace that what had happened, happened. I could not change it. I could not move back the clock to days earlier. My brother was no longer on earth, but he was with the Lord. And with that realization, I was able to start working through my grief and bring an end to my days of mourning.

Since that time, I have lost other close friends and relatives. None of these passings has been easy to take, but each has brought me closer to God. I see his hand in life, as well as death, in my own faith walk, and in the faces and hearts of others. I am more comforted by my own sense of mortality, too, because I see how God works through each of us to bring us along and lead us gently home.

I know that his promise of the Resurrection is for me and my brothers and sisters in Christ—and for that gift, I rejoice!

There is no doubt that coping with the death of a loved one when you yourself suffer from serious illness brings a certain unique set of problems. You must make sure that, even as you tend to the "business" of a death, you tend to your own health needs. You must comfort others *and* reach out for comfort for yourself. And you must come closer to God at a time when you might feel most abandoned by him, or betrayed.

The more time you allow yourself to work through your grief, to acknowledge the darkness and seek the light, the more you will feel lifted up by the Lord. And the more you seek his healing of heart and soul, the more deeply you will be cleansed and made fresh, living a new and sparkling life in light of his Salvation.

O Lord, I am torn up with grief.
I know you are there, but I cannot see past
my sorrow and tears.
Be with me, Lord, and do not take
my unhappiness to heart.
Rather, work within me to guide me through
these dark days
and bring your light to my life,
so that I may see your goodness, even in my mourning.

GIVING UP

For just as the sufferings of Christ flow over into our lives, so also through Christ our comfort overflows. If we are distressed, it is for your comfort and salvation; if we are comforted, it is for your comfort, which produces in you patient endurance of the same sufferings we suffer. And our hope for you is firm, because we know that just as you share in our sufferings, so also you share in our comfort.
—*2 Corinthians 1:5–7, New International Version*

Each day, each step along the path of having a serious illness brings challenges. And just when you think you're over the "worst," something else comes up. The insurance company denies your claim for treatment. Blood tests come back indicating a complication. Your child has a breakdown because she's afraid "Mommy's going to die." Your boss tells you he can't shoulder the burden of your increased absences and says you must decide between your job and your health. . . .

Each of these situations by itself would probably be workable. But you are not in the best of health, and these stresses weigh upon you with ever-increasing burden. If one straw can break the camel's back, think of what all of these problems are doing to yours!

Sometimes you feel like giving up.

All around the world at this very moment, there are others like you, people suffering excruciating pain and wondering if they have the stamina to continue living. There are people for whom the simplest daily chore is beyond their capability—and they feel like giving up on ever living a "normal" life again. Closer to home, someone is sitting in a darkened room, crying in frustration at all of life's burdens.

But just as there are others on the brink of giving up, there are people who have stood at the edge of the same precipice and found a way to move back from it. People have overcome tremendous obstacles and discovered a way to be hopeful and move through the trials and into a new kind of strength and light. Their examples are inspirations for those of us who despair, and they are also comforting. For if other people have faced the same hardships as you have and moved beyond them to find inner strength and endurance, you can do the same.

Throughout the Bible are stories of valiant men and women living through plagues and storms, inner doubt and external scourges. Their triumphs are learning tools for us; through them, we can find sustenance for our journey through the "desert," and prayers for our souls, too. In our neighborhoods, in our towns, and throughout the world, there are living examples of resilience and courage that we can learn from, too, and take to heart. How much better can it be, to learn about the journey from others who have been there?

There is a seamless circle and a flow to the reading above from Corinthians, and it reflects the endless ways that we are bound with our fellow sufferers and held up by them and for them. We are not all at the same place in our journey with illness, but through our suffering, we can be brought closer to others in fellowship and trust. And through our times of comfort and victory over adversity, we can be inspirational for others who are at lower points in their walk. It is part of our responsibility and our calling to not give up, but rather to continue in the circle of fellowship, being held up and holding up, in turn, among our beloved brothers and sisters.

Seeing your illness in the context of a whole community of sufferers and learning from the experiences of others can bring remarkable calm and comfort to you in your time of trial. You do not need to give up, for there is a way through the difficult time you have right now. Others have done it. They, and the Lord, are with you. And with you firmly in their hands and hearts, you will walk safely through the fire and reach the other side.

O Lord, I am on the brink of giving up.
But I know that you will make a way for me
to continue.
I am feeling so very alone.
But I know that you have placed me among a
remarkable fellowship of others
who have lived through similar times.
Please help me take up full membership in the circle
of believers
and learn from them, and you, about how I can act,
so that I do not give up, but rather move through
this time
and on to the promises you most assuredly have made
for me.

LIVING TRUE TO GOD

For we speak as messengers who have been approved by God to be
entrusted with the Good News. Our purpose is to please God, not
people. He is the one who examines the motives of our hearts.
—*1 Thessalonians 2:4, New Living Translation*

In your life with illness, you will face many decisions about
how to handle your condition. You will need to work with
your doctor and your family, to a certain extent, on just what
you will do or not do regarding treatment, second opinions,
and lifestyle changes. But the ultimate decisions will be yours,
and sometimes you will be going against the wishes of others.

For this reason, a vibrant prayer life, where you are close to
God and intent upon listening to his will for you, is essential
to finding peace with the decisions you make and the conse-
quences of them. For example, if you have been diagnosed
with cancer and are facing the decision about whether or not
to go through surgery and long courses of chemotherapy
and/or radiation treatment, external pressures might be tremendous. Your family might want you to undergo these treatments, to prolong your life as much as possible even if your
quality of life will not be the best. Your doctor might try to
convince you that you need extra treatments or new therapies,
but might not give you enough assurance that they will bring
the desired results. But even in the face of all of these pres-

sures, you are, ultimately, the one who has to undergo the procedures or let the disease take its course.

You are the one who must make these decisions. And it is only through close communion with the Lord that you will be able to reach calm and peace with what you decide to do.

If you are living with a less life-threatening illness, you will also have to make decisions about what is best for your health. If you have lupus, for example, how much sun exposure you get is up to you; even if you are persuaded by loved ones that "one hour shouldn't hurt," you must have the inner strength to resist them if sun sensitivity is a factor in the severity of your disease. If you have diabetes, you will need to make decisions about your diet every day and resist societal pressures to eat foods that might not be good for you.

Perhaps you feel weakened because of pain or worn down because of the constant struggle of living with a serious illness. Perhaps you don't think you have the fortitude to see your health challenge through and want to leave crucial decisions up to others.

Lift up your concerns and your weakness to the Lord. He will give you all that you need to do, and say what is right for you, what is strong and true. He will not forsake you, no matter how dire your circumstances. And he will give you wisdom to respond to all of the many situations you will find yourself in to make decisions that are life-bringing and healthy for you.

The Lord has given us our bodies and our lives, creating us in his image and expecting us to take good care of ourselves. Each day we will come in contact with people and things that would sway us from what is ultimately good and dignifying for us.

Living true to God means making decisions that might go against what others would want us to do. It means being close to God and acting in a way that gives glory to his creation of our bodies and our lives. It means living in *his* will and *his* truth, no matter what anyone else says.

> *Lord, my God, I am beset by confusion over*
> *what is best to decide.*
> *Troubled as I am, I want to do only what is right*
> *and what is true to you.*
> *Please help me to act and speak in a way*
> *that is pleasing to you,*
> *and let me make decisions that protect and keep*
> *this wonderful creation you have given me,*
> *this body . . .*
> *this life.*

DO YOU WORRY THAT GOD
WILL ABANDON YOU?

And at the ninth hour, Jesus cried out in a loud voice, "Eloi, Eloi, lama sabachthani?"—which means, "My God, my God, why have you forsaken me?"

—Mark 15:34, New International Version

Do you ever worry that God will tire of you and your illness? Do you ever worry that you will reach a point where the Lord will say "Enough" and leave you? Abandon you?

Jesus' cry "at the ninth hour" is very powerful. After his life of travel, witness, and persecution, the long walk up to Calvary, and the excruciating crucifixion, his question to God rings with urgency and frustration with a stark humanity that moves me to my soul. After all that Jesus has done and suffered, his human-centered worst fear is realized: he feels that God has abandoned him.

But although Jesus' moment was dark, indeed, in his humanity, he could not see (or at least did not express) the glory that would come after his death. Rather than being abandoned by God, Jesus was being taken through the "desert" to rise again, to fulfill his human journey and be joined with his Father. Yes, no matter how much despair Jesus felt just before his death, God never abandoned him.

And, no matter how much pain and suffering we go through, God never abandons us, either.

To better understand the unlimited scope and power of God's love, we can turn first to our experience with human love. Sometimes even the strongest bonds will be shaken because one person in the relationship changes or troubles become too overwhelming for love to endure. Other times our loved one might do something that breaks the trust and respect that we had held previously; when this happens, love can wither and die quickly and be impossible to revive.

Our experience of friendships shows us that they, too, can be breakable, or at least fluid. Time passes. People move away. Priorities intervene. Friendships ebb and flow.

Each of us has experienced abandonment by a loved one at least once in our life with illness. From our own experience, our fear that certain people, be they friends or relatives, will turn away from us is quite natural. We worry that we might be too much of a "burden" for them or that they will get "tired" of our complaining. But our relationship with the Lord is quite different from any we will have with another human being.

The Lord created each of us in his image and gives us our lives.

The Lord gives us wonderful miracles each day and night.

The Lord gives us his eternal salvation!

If we reflect on each of the many things God gives us, we can't help but wonder at his love and abiding presence. Through good times and bad, the Lord sustains us, just as he did his Son.

If God brought Jesus through the wilderness, as our most perfect example, and did not abandon him, how can we believe God will ever abandon us? Yes, our road is long. There will be times when we might not think God is as close to us as we would like. There will be times, too, when we will cry out to God, asking him "Why have you abandoned me?"

But even as we cry out, God is with us each step, just as he was with his Son each painful stride to Calvary and all through the anguishing moments of his crucifixion.

Jesus' cry demonstrates his utter humanity at the most painful, lonely moment in his life. But underneath his suffering was hope, borne of God's promise and power.

May this give us comfort, too, when we cry out, that God will never abandon us.

He loves us completely and forever.

O Lord, at times I feel as though you must be so tired of
my complaining!
If my friends and loved ones heard all of my prayers,
they'd certainly turn away!
Help me to know, deep within, that you are
ever with me.
No matter how loudly I cry to you,
please know that I love you completely and forever,
just as you love me.

JOY THAT RUNNETH OVER

So, my dear brothers and sisters, be strong and steady, always enthusiastic about the Lord's work, for you know that nothing you do
for the Lord is ever useless.
    —*1 Corinthians 15:58, New Living Translation*

Mundane activities do not naturally give me a "spiritual
high." After all, doesn't it sound a little ridiculous to
shout, "Praise you God for my new can opener!" or "What a
wonderful day God has made! I moved my big toe!"? Some
things on the face of them do not engender my greatest enthusiasm, either. I am not exactly bubbling over with mirth as
I pay for my monthly prescriptions or ask the phlebotomist
to use a butterfly when drawing my blood. Yet, in the face of
the most routine (and sometimes painful) situations, I am
reminded of this reading from Corinthians: ". . . be strong
and steady, always enthusiastic about the Lord's work." That
phrase and the next one, ". . . nothing you do for the Lord is
ever useless," ring loudly with the importance of treasuring
each gift God gives us and *everything* he gives us to do with unbridled appreciation, with joy that runneth over. My own experience is a testimony to this, too. (Isn't it just the way that we
often forget what is most important to remember?)

When I was diagnosed with lupus, I did not even know
what it was. I assumed there would be medication to "cure" it

and readily available information about the disease and coping with it. Very quickly I learned how wrong I was. First of all, there is no cure for lupus, and treating it is extremely difficult and frustrating (for the patient and, I'm sure, for the doctor). Second, the information I found in those early days was either very technical or very scary (some of it assumed that lupus patients would live a maximum of five years after diagnosis, and that was all).

As I began treatment, I also began a "lupus journal," which I intended for my eyes (and God's eyes) only. I also began gathering information about lupus. I was steady about taking my medication and reading up on the disease. And I was strong about my conviction that there should be something better for us "lupies." But I never thought that my very "usual" activities would lead to writing a book about lupus, let alone getting it published and distributed to other patients!

Each thing that I did to manage my disease gave me some knowledge and insight that found their way into the book. And, with each step toward publication, I experienced an amazing joy and awe at what God was doing in my life. Even the very "tiny" things, such as buying an arthritis-friendly pen, brought me closer to the finished work and more deeply sure that God's hand was in the large things as well as the small. He was and still is in full control.

My joy runneth over!

Since finishing *Taking Charge of Lupus*, I have been given the opportunity to write other books, including this one. Each has taken me on a remarkable journey of discovery, especially in the "small things." And each is full of surprises and revelation that I can only praise God for.

We never know what impact our actions and words will have on others, and we never know where our travel with serious illness will lead. But we do know that if we embrace the totality of our lives with *joy that runneth over*, we will be given fulfilling work on earth and a treasure beyond compare in heaven.

O Lord, I sometimes get bored with the small things
in my life.
Please open my eyes to the simple wonders
all around me.
Help me appreciate them, too,
with strong and steady enthusiasm.
And witness to you in everything
with joy that runneth over.

You Matter

There is no word or sound,
no voice heard,
Yet their report goes forth through all the earth,
their message, to the ends of the world.
—*Psalm 19:4–5, New American Bible*

As you explore the new world of living with a serious illness, you will probably find out about organizations that are dedicated to providing patient services, research, and information about your condition. There might be advertisements about drugs targeted at your illness, or word of new treatments. You might turn on the radio and hear a public service announcement about your condition or see a telethon broadcast nationwide. Government agencies will issue reports based on statistics of how many people have what you have and break down the numbers demographically according to geographic area, ethnicity, sex, and mortality.

With limited resources, energy, and money, you might wonder if there is any way you can become involved in promoting awareness and research about your illness. You might think you are only a number to the medical community in general (and perhaps to your doctor, too), and you might ask yourself (as I did), "Do I matter in this world of sickness? And if so, how?"

If you feel small in the medical community, you also might feel insignificant in the world at large, especially if you are not able to be as productive or active as you once were. Again, this might cause you to wonder, "Do I matter? If so, how?"

Although there are billions of other people on the planet at any given time, God knows each by name. Even more, he can count the hairs on each head, hear the prayers of each supplicant, and answer each plea individually. What an awesome God we serve!

We see the effect of something small on a large whole all around us. Observe the beauty of nature—and how each plant and animal combines to make that wonderful picture. Hear the majesty of a lush symphony, a brilliant combination of many smaller parts. Feel the smoothness of a favorite sweater and think of all the hands that worked on various stages of it to bring it to where it is now.

In your own life, the small things you do add up to a very complete whole. Each movement you make enables you to proceed through the day. Each word you say adds up to whole sentences and thoughts. Your various actions impact others, too, sometimes in ways you don't expect. Think of all the times someone has said, "I'm glad you said that. I needed to hear it," or you surprised someone in an uplifting way.

Your presence is vital to the happiness of many people, and it can even enhance the lives of strangers whom you've never met. The parking attendant who tells you how much you owe . . . the postal worker who delivers your mail . . . the person at church who just joined the congregation . . . each of these people will benefit from a kind word or smile from you. In fact, you can make their day!

When we realize that no task we take on, no sound we make, will not go unheard or unfelt, we can begin to find our place in the world around us with more confidence. We can also have faith that we will make a difference, a positive difference, in that world. You do not have to think of finding a cure for muscular dystrophy, for example, but you can talk with a newly diagnosed patient and share your experience.

Reflecting on how much we truly do impact others can be a humbling task. If I consider how my words and actions affect others and reach up to my Lord, I am much more inclined to think before I speak or perform any task. Yet the room for doing good far outweighs the room for committing error. After all, we can't keep our light under a bushel!

Do you matter? Do I? The Lord knows we do. And as we go through our lives from this time forward, aware of the import of that fact, our insignificance will, itself, seem insignificant, and we will behave and feel as we truly are: Beloved children of God and lights for this world.

O Lord, you are far greater than anything or anyone
I could ever know.
Help me to feel your power work through me,
and in all of my activities, in all of what I say,
let me reflect your light and bring your help
in great ways,
if it is your will,
and small.

JESUS IN THE GARDEN

[Jesus] said, "Abba, Father, all things are possible to you. Take this cup away from me, but not what I will, but what you will."
—*Mark 14:36, New American Bible*

Watching springtime bulbs burst forth from the earth in our gardens and shoot up to the sky, becoming bright green leaves and brilliant flowers, is one of the joys of moving from winter into warmer, sunnier times. It is also a very real witness to the kind of spiritual transformation that Jesus experienced in his garden on the eve of his apprehension, trial, and crucifixion, and the kind of development we go through as we release our human fears and desires and fully accept God's will for our lives.

Indeed, releasing the control that we have over our lives and letting God take over is one of the most difficult yet holy things we could ever do. It requires all of our faith and trust, and much courage, too. And, rather than being confining, it is above all things completely freeing. As we see in the above reading from Mark, Jesus' example of accepting his Father's will is not devoid of human longing for avoidance of the suffering and pain he was to undergo. He acknowledges God's omnipotence and asks for "this cup" to be taken away. But in the same breath, he puts himself under God's total guidance. He tells God that he wants not his own will but the Lord's will to be done. In subjugating himself before the Father, he goes through hell on earth to achieve a forever heaven—he rises from the earth to become a glorious flower.

Arriving at the point of complete yielding to God's will in a life filled with illness, frustration, and yearning for something better is not easy. The more ill you are, the more you want to be healthy. The more pain you feel, the more relief you crave. Each step along the path of sickness makes you want to run away, not trudge ahead into more hardship. Yet this longing to be anywhere but where you are is the human side of being seriously ill. This longing is a heavy burden that stands in the way of your coming to peace with your illness and being ready to do whatever God ordains for you. Your human hesitation is, in a very real way, what holds you back from being a full child of God.

Much like the plants that grew there, Jesus started off his time in prayer rooted in the earth of his humanity, giving the power to God, and asking that his suffering be taken from him. But in a wonderful manifestation of spiritual growth, Jesus then lifted himself upward, reached toward the heavens, and came to the point where his humanity was under God's command. No longer was he bound by his humanity. He was on a higher, more holy path.

To become the people God means for us to be, we too must be conscious of opportunities to let ourselves blossom in faith. We must push the confining earth away from ourselves and reach for the heavens, for the warmth of God's love and the light of his presence. We must accept also rain and troubles as a natural, nurturing part of our growth. We must open ourselves to all of God's possibilities for our lives—and leave behind all that would separate ourselves from him.

It is a miracle to me that tulip, daffodil, crocus, and lily of the valley bulbs can weather stormy, frigid winters and still rise to gorgeous life when spring warms the earth. In the same way, it is amazing to me how much we can truly endure in the way of hardship and still reflect the awesomeness of God's creation. It is also wonderful to think that helping our faith grow shows others what our God can do, just as seeing those early blossoms signals the end to a hard winter and the beginning of new life and new hope.

When you are most in despair, when you most want to turn away from what God is leading you to, then is the time to acknowledge your humanness and ask God for the faith and courage to go on, in his light, in his way. No matter how deep your winter may be, he will lead you through to a glorious spring.

O Lord, I am in such anguish that I wish this cup
could be taken away.
But, at the same time, I know that you have a glorious
future planned for me.
Help me to bend myself to your will, now and always,
and let me blossom forth from this harsh earth
and become the shining witness
that you mean for me to be.

ARE YOU WAITING
FOR A MIRACLE?

[Abel . . . Enoch . . . Noah . . . Abraham . . .] All these people were
still living by faith when they died. They did not receive the things
promised; they only saw them and welcomed them from a distance.
And they admitted that they were aliens and strangers on earth.
People who say such things show that they are looking for a country of their own. If they had been thinking of the country they had
left, they would have had opportunity to return. Instead, they were
longing for a better country—a heavenly one. Therefore, God is not
ashamed to be called their God, for he has prepared a city for them.
—*Hebrews 11:13–16, New International Version*

There is a very familiar story about the man whose house
was surrounded by floodwaters. He went to the top of the
roof and prayed for God to rescue him. Three times, people in
boats came by and offered their assistance. Three times, the
man told them he was waiting on the Lord.

Finally the floodwaters engulfed the house completely and
the man drowned.

When the man reached heaven, he said to God, "Lord, I
prayed to you for your miracle to save me. Why didn't you answer my prayer?"

God replied, "I sent you three boats. What more did you
want?"

. . .

How many times in your life have you "waited for a miracle," a bolt of lightning from the sky or some other divine intervention to save you from a particularly difficult situation?

How many times have you prayed for God to "save you," but haven't recognized his hand in the assistance offered by human means?

When we are seriously ill, it is very human to pray for God to take away our suffering, to cure us completely. We know that God has the power to do this, and we have heard of examples where he has done just this for others. But it is unreasonable to think that in all cases, God will work a miracle "solo."

Sometimes he works through other people.

Sometimes he works through the medication we must take.

Sometimes he works through the things that we do to make ourselves feel better.

We can never ignore the importance of doing all we can do to help ourselves be healthier. Our bodies are gifts from God, and we have a responsibility to take good care of them. So, if we develop unhealthful habits, we cannot then be angry that God hasn't "cured" us. First we must learn good health habits.

Also vital is keeping our souls and emotional lives healthy. God *can* cure us. But if we *expect* him to simply give us back our health, we are overlooking the duty we have to him, the obedience we must give him.

The people mentioned in the reading from Hebrews "were still living by faith when they died." It is a testimony to their faith that "they did not receive the things promised" before they passed on. It is also a testimony to God that he made a way for them through their earthly lives and bestowed his gift upon them when they finally died, a "heavenly" country.

If Noah had not built the ark, would he have survived the flood?

If Moses had not defied Pharaoh, would the Israelites have been freed?

If Jesus had not lived his life on earth, would the Salvation he brought have meant the same as it does?

If we don't do our part and take up our responsibility as children of God, will we be recipients of a miracle?

It is a question worth pondering.

Yes, God can work wonders.

But just as important is how we live in the meantime.

O Lord, help me to help you work in my life.
Let me not take your graciousness and gifts for granted.
Let me keep my hands busy and my spirit alive,
so that I may take care of all that you give me,
and be worthy of your goodness.

FACING DISABILITY

Three times I begged the Lord about this, that it might leave me, but he said to me, "My grace is sufficient for you, for power is made perfect in weakness." I will rather boast most gladly of my weaknesses in order that the power of Christ may dwell in me.
—*2 Corinthians 12:8–9, New American Bible*

For many people, the word "disability" is very difficult to say, let alone associate with themselves personally. Some even put off applying for disability insurance benefits because they do not want to be "labeled" with such a negative word. In recent years there have been phrases that substitute for it: "Physically challenged." "Differently abled." "Otherwise abled." But the meaning is still clear, and so is the stigma. The "disabled" are often lumped into the "needy" category by society or looked at with some degree of scorn, especially if groups representing disabled people sue corporations or otherwise try to assert certain rights.

If you are on the verge of applying for disability status or have recently done so, you might find the adjustment to your new "title" hard to take. To you, being disabled might mean that you are giving up the fight to be productive, that you have lost the race, that you are no longer a valid member of the human community. Although your status might open up financial and medical resources, it might also seem to close doors;

explaining to a new love interest that you are "disabled" might cause that person to turn away rather than pursue the relationship. And if you decide to apply for a job, even part-time, having to tell a potential employer that you have been disabled might be a mark against you in the hiring process.

In your own heart and soul, it is important to make the distinction between what being disabled means on paper and what it means in your life. You could very well be physically disabled but still find ways to be productive and contributing to the world around you. You might draw your financial support from disability resources, but after all, you have paid into them during your working years. If applying for disability will allow you access to certain privileges (such as a special parking permit), and your health will benefit from them, there is nothing wrong with going through the application procedure if you qualify.

Above all, no matter what titles we might have gone by prior to becoming ill, they are nothing compared with the truth that lies within each of us as children of God, the "grace" that the Lord gives us. This reality is more important and more precious than any of the man-made categories that we might find ourselves in, and it is certainly more useful when looking at who we are and where we fit into God's creation.

Denying our physical constraints, our "disabilities," can work against us as we strive to be witnesses to God. As Paul says in this reading from Corinthians, "I will rather boast most gladly of my weaknesses in order that the power of Christ may dwell in me." Your physical condition is a real presence in your life, but so is the Lord. It is through you, even in your weakness, that he can work amazing wonders:

"Power is made perfect in weakness."

You might encounter resistance from family and friends when you tell them you are going on disability. They, too, might have reservations about what kinds of doors will close for you and what implications the "title" will mean to your emotional and societal status. But what a wonderful opportunity this is to witness to how God is working in you and through you. What a way to show others that you are accepting of his plan for your life!

As with all of the challenges you have faced and overcome thus far, facing disability is yet another step in fulfilling God's plan for you. As his grace fills you abundantly, know that no matter what society may say you are, in his eyes, you are, as his child, fully and powerfully abled!

O Lord, help me to be patient and understanding
with myself and others
as I go through the disability process.
Lead me through the paperwork and processes
so that I may fulfill your plan for me
and continue to do what is right, just, and good.

FORCED TO RELY ON OTHERS

Is any one of you sick? He should call the elders of the church to
pray over him and anoint him with oil in the name of the Lord. And
the prayer offered in faith will make the sick person well; the Lord
will raise him up. If he has sinned, he will be forgiven.

—*James 5:14–15, New International Version*

We might feel very alone as we proceed through our lives
of illness. But we cannot overlook the importance of relying upon others in a very proactive and spirit-filled way. In
our church community and beyond, we need to be mindful of
the role that our fellow Christians can exercise and the way
God can work through them, just as he works through us.

Relying on others can give us support in ways we can't begin to imagine. It can also bring us closer to God.

Oh, reliance upon others has its human side, too. There
are the friends who insist they will "do anything" for you, but
when asked they don't seem to have the time. There are others who want to rush in and take over the whole situation,
down to what kind of sheets you have on your sickbed. Still
others will agree to take you to an appointment, and then be so
late that your nerves are frazzled and you feel as though you
would have been better off not asking them at all.

Even in prayer, others can act in a way that is contrary to
what you think you want—or need. They might pray that you

fully recover from your illness, only to be disappointed when you don't. They might look at you with expectant eyes, as though you will be completely transformed in their presence. They might even hint (or say outright) that you are doing something to "stand in the way" of answers to their prayers— a sure sign that they are not exactly on the same spiritual page as you are!

But for all the foibles and failings of others, their help is vital to each of us, and the support of loved ones is immeasurably important. Especially in prayer, when you are lifted up by others, you are truly a participant in the God-given directive: "Love one another."

I participate in a number of formal and informal prayer-centered groups. We ask for prayers for specific things and also for general comfort. Sometimes I cannot pinpoint the exact moment when a prayer has been answered; however, I know that the overwhelming outpouring of spirit that comes from each moment in collective prayer can only help others and me to grow.

In the same way, when I have asked for others to pray for me, the extent of blessing and grace can bring a feeling of wellness that surpasses a physical cure. Even if my symptoms do not subside, I am better for having prayer lifted up on my behalf.

The Lord truly does "raise me up."

And even more blessed, I know my sins are forgiven.

As we live through the lonely days and nights, isolated in pain and suffering, let's not forget that we need each other to pray, if not to physically help. We might not know each other by name, we might never meet. But I know that I feel immensely better as part of the circle of believers than I do without, and I thrive upon fellowship of my brothers and sisters, even if my illness does not go away.

At any given time, one of us will be sick. Reflect upon that.

Think of the healing that God brings to each of us. Pour out your heart to everyone who needs comfort and solace. Pray for all throughout the world who suffer and are sad.

And I will pray for you.

O Lord, I rejoice at the fellowship of my
brothers and sisters in faith.
Please let me not hesitate to call upon them,
but rather welcome their help, physical and spiritual,
into my life.
That I, in turn, might be of help to them,
whenever they might need me.

Mourning the Loss
of Health

No, dear brothers and sisters, I am still not all I should be, but I am
focusing all my energies on this one thing: Forgetting the past and
looking forward to what lies ahead. I strain to reach the end of the
race and receive the prize for which God, through Christ Jesus, is
calling us up to heaven.

—*Philippians 3:13–14, New Living Translation*

There are many stages to mourning the loss of someone
you love, including denial, anger, bargaining, and final acceptance. Working through these stages is very important to
moving into and past grief, but individuals do not go through
them at the same pace, nor do they follow in a specific se-
quential order. In much the same way, you grieve the loss of
your health when you are diagnosed with a serious illness. And
you must work through the stages of that grieving so that you
can achieve acceptance and progress in faith and well-being.

Although I am well beyond the early stages of my diagnosis and treatment with lupus, there are still times when I feel
anger, denial, or other emotions associated with the grieving
process. Meditating on my emotional and spiritual status at
any given time helps me determine where I am in regard to my
grief and acceptance. So, too, does prayer in which I speak little but listen deeply to what God is telling me.

Little things will trigger my awareness that I am still, in some way, grieving. A picture from a vacation pre-lupus will remind me of the sunshine I can no longer enjoy. A song on the radio will recall a more pain-free time. There are still people I know from previous jobs and college who don't know I have lupus; explaining my diagnosis and what it means to my life brings up all those old feelings once again.

On a very good day, I might forget that I have lupus and forge ahead through all kinds of activities, only to be exhausted and achy the next day. When this happens I feel stymied, like a spirited horse being restrained by a firm-handed rider, and I mourn the loss of feeling the proverbial wind in my face.

I can truly identify with Paul when he says, "No, dear brothers and sisters, I am still not all I should be." I *feel* I should be all over with mourning the loss of my health. But then something will trigger a memory . . . and I'll go back over the same territory all over again.

Paul recognizes this tendency. He experienced it himself. He says, "I am focusing all my energies on this one thing: Forgetting the past and looking forward to what lies ahead." What a great reminder that our goal is not here on earth, but at the "end of the race," in heaven!

Indeed, our lives are full of losses, not just of health but of loved ones and opportunities. Even if we were to age in perfect health, there would still be things we would lose—hair, teeth, the suppleness of our skin, our "girlish" or "manly" physiques. I suppose you could say that while we live on earth, we will lose . . . but so that we may receive the ultimate prize with God.

Sometimes I joke with my healthy friends and tell them that I'm going through all of this arthritis and other physical problems so that I can be well prepared for old age. I tell them that all of the losses I'm going through put me in a perfect position to give them pointers when they "get there."

In some ways, I will. But in other ways, I know that I'm only human. My emotions will sometimes get the better of me and I'll be "set back" to work through, again, part of my mourning process. I understand that. I'm not angry about it. I don't fight it. But I also try to keep Paul's words in my mind and heart. I strive to not focus so much on my losses, but rather keep my "eyes on the prize," so that even in my lowest moments I can feel the hope and comfort of God's promise—and my eternal gain.

O Lord, bring me through my mourning
with a deeper sense of comfort and peace.
Help me understand that I might feel grief about losing
my health for a long time,
but that you hold for me a prize surpassing all others,
a calling for me in heaven that will eclipse any loss
I may ever sustain.

COPING WITH FATIGUE

How long, O sluggard, will you rest?
When will you rise from your sleep?
—*Proverbs 6:9, New American Bible*

"I have lupus?" I asked.

"Yes," replied my rheumatologist.

"And one of the symptoms is fatigue? Really, really horrible fatigue?"

"Yes."

"How do I deal with it? What should I do?"

"You have to rest. You have to take naps and get a lot of sleep at other times, too."

"ALL RIGHT!" I yelled.

My rheumatologist was shocked. "What?!"

"I have permission to sleep!"

Since I was a teenager and clocked about fifteen to sixteen hours of sleep a night, I have always required a lot of rest, a lot of "downtime." The year before I was diagnosed with lupus, I was especially fatigued. Even when I got a lot of sleep, I could barely get through a day without feeling as if I could nod off wherever I was—in the middle of the supermarket, while driving, in a meeting.

To be told I had lupus was terrible, of course. But to be given permission to sleep, to be *told* by my doctor that I *had* to rest, nap, and sleep, well, to me this was and still is a gift directly from the Lord.

And yet, not everyone shared my jubilation. I couldn't work any longer at a "steady" job—not many employers allow employees to take multiple naps. I often had to cancel social engagements at the last minute because I was simply too tired. Some of my loved ones assumed that eight hours was ample sleep and barely disguised their skepticism that I *really* needed more rest than that. Or people wondered after a few months or years if I was "finally over that sleep thing."

I have to admit that I, too, became irritated if I had to stop doing something enjoyable or cut short a visit with a friend because I couldn't keep my eyes open. In fact, the reading above from Proverbs echoes how I sometimes talk to myself. Sometimes not even *I* believe I need as much rest as I do.

But I do.

And as the realization of that has become more ingrained in me, I have learned that sleep is like any other medication and brings benefits that cannot be contained in a pill or inhaler. It rejuvenates, revives, and nourishes us. We, as people with serious illness, need to be sure we get enough of it. This might mean going against the wishes of your loved ones or disappointing them because you cannot be as active as they want you to be. But your first responsibility is to make sure you do all that you can for yourself to help your health and promote your well-being.

There is another kind of sleep, however, that is not as beneficial as physical rest. That is the sleep of the soul. We should always be wakeful when it comes to our spiritual selves, and always be alert to the Lord's work in our lives. In that regard, the reading from Proverbs applies, too. I suppose I can say that we need to be spiritually and emotionally awake to the fact that we need physical sleep!

We can support our need for sleep by creating living environments that are conducive to rest and by making sure we allow the time to prepare for bed and relaxation. Just as important, we can keep ourselves awake to our physical and spiritual needs, and always respond to what God is telling us to do, what he wants us to do to take care of these lives he has given us.

O Lord, even as I sleep, keep my soul awake to you.
Help me to be still and quiet, letting sleep fall
upon my body
so that I may be refreshed and ever ready
to live the kind of life
you would have me live.

FEAR OF TRAVELING

"With unfailing love you will lead this people whom you have ransomed.
You will guide them in your strength, to the place where your
holiness dwells."
—*Exodus 15:13, New Living Translation*

It might seem impossible to think of traveling if you suffer from a serious illness. Especially in today's world, the act of going afar, from place to place, can be extremely difficult. But as daunting as the thought of boarding an airplane, ship, or train might be, there can sometimes be no substitute for being present in a new place or visiting far-flung loved ones.

How can you allay your fears about traveling? How can you make your journey as comfortable and safe as possible?

Taking physical precautions is, of course, very important. You need to be sure that traveling will not aggravate your health condition, and you also need to account for all the treatment and medical issues you have to take care of. Just as vital to making your journey a good one is, however, preparing yourself spiritually and emotionally. God's hand is in all that you are and all that you do. He is with you, too, on any trip you might undertake.

Your faith brings you through the darkest of moments at home. Through prayer and meditations, you endure long medical examinations, tests, and medication regimens. You rely on God's steadying hand to bolster your courage at such times, and you know that he is working within you and those around you, no matter what the circumstances. In the same way, the hope and faith you have in God should be the first thing that you "pack" when preparing for a trip. It is in a very real sense your "ticket" to making it through the hard hours of traveling, and it is what will lead you to comfort, rest, and home at journey's end.

God's presence has been with many travelers throughout time. He accompanied the Israelites and paved the way for them to reach the Promised Land. He protected Mary, Joseph, and the baby Jesus as they fled Herod's persecution and arrived in exile in Egypt. He walked each dusty step with the adult Jesus and the apostles, who reached the far-off corners of their known world.

Although many biblical travelers did not have an easy time of their journeying, God still held them up and led them through. Through the Red Sea. Through the desert. Through storms. Through crowds of angry unbelievers. He fed them with manna, multiplied fishes, brought restful sleep to the weary.

And he led them all home.

The sweetness of greeting loved ones you haven't seen in a long while, the awe of seeing natural and man-made wonders in distant lands, and the act of stretching yourself physically and mentally are joyful benefits of arriving at your journey's end. It might take extra effort on your part to make sure that pretrip preparations allow for all of your physical needs on the way, but all of your work will be worth it as you reap the rewards of travel. And with all that you gain from venturing out of your known and comfortable world, you will learn even more about God's presence in your life and his purpose for you.

Yes, traveling can be daunting, fearsome, even seemingly

impossible. But if it is something that, after much prayer and reflection, you feel you are being led to do, then God will make a way for you.

He did it for the Israelites.

He did it for the holy family.

He did it for the apostles.

He did it for the missionaries of days past and present.

And he will do it for you, too. And be with you every step of the way.

Lord Jesus, give me the courage to face my journey
as part of my walk with you.
Take away my fear and replace it with resolve
to plan my travel wisely and approach it
enthusiastically.
For no matter where you lead me,
I know that you will bring me home.

VISUALIZING GOOD HEALTH

Who is this that appears like the dawn,
fair as the moon,
bright as the sun, majestic as the stars in procession?
—*The Song of Songs 6:10, New International Version*

Think of yourself at your healthiest, "bright as the sun, majestic as the stars." You have no pain, no sorrow. All of your internal organs function perfectly and your outward appearance is radiant and joyful. Your movements are youthful. Your laughter is contagious. Your eyes look at the world with fresh insight. Your tongue speaks the praises of God and the awe that you feel about simply being alive.

This act of visualizing yourself in full health is a very important part of encouraging yourself to attain as healthful a state as you possibly can, but it is often something you do not do because it seems so impossible. If you have been sick for a long while, you might have forgotten what it is like to feel healthy. If your physical condition is deteriorating, you might not believe that it can ever get better, so you might think, "What's the use in dreaming?"

Yet the same technique used by high achievers in many walks of life, including successful athletes, businesspeople, and artists, is something that we can also use, and to very good benefit. After all, if visualizing heaven leads us to conduct ourselves in better, more Godlike ways, won't visualizing good health give us more hope for feeling and functioning better, too?

As Christians, we have our "eyes on the prize" both day and night. We know that the Lord has a wonderful eternal life prepared for us, and the promise of his Salvation is unquestionable. We yearn for heaven, long for it, plan for it. We cannot see it on this earth, we will not experience it until we die, and yet we believe in its reality and let our belief affect how we act, what we say, and why we move on through hardships.

In the same way, by visualizing health, we encourage ourselves to adopt better habits and activities that will enhance our physical states. We become more positive in how we view our lives and we give our course of treatment more of an opportunity to work because of this. In our thoughts and prayers, if we focus on being more healthful, the Lord will lead us to ways to be just that. He might not bring us a full cure, but he will bring us a better sense of well-being.

Today's scientists have just begun studies of the effects of positive visualization upon medical treatments. There is some evidence that approaching a specific treatment, say, radiation therapy, with a positive attitude can make the treatment more effective than it would be if the patient did not believe there was any chance of its working. Likewise, patients who were given medication and who believed it would not work had a higher incidence of experiencing just that.

All scientific studies aside, we know that if we approach our lives positively and in faith, we are better equipped to overcome obstacles. Spiritually, if you approach your healthcare with a pessimistic attitude of "it'll never work," if you cling to the credo "I'll never be better," then it is more likely that this is what will happen. But if you reach for good health like you reach for heaven, you will be filled with an optimism that can boost your spirits and bring you insight about what, in the ideal world, can be.

Heaven.

Health.

These are things we strive for. If we didn't keep the best of these in mind and heart, our lives would be very dark indeed. But because we are children of the light, beloved by God, we know that heaven is within our reach. By visualizing health, we give ourselves the image of wholeness that can inspire us to a better, stronger way of living:

"Who is this that appears like the day, fair as the moon, bright as the sun?"

Could it be you?

O Lord, I find it hard to remember what it was like
to be healthy.
Help me keep my mind focused on good health
and strength.
Let me be positive about the course of treatment
I am undergoing.
And let me always have faith, great faith,
in your presence in my life
and your glory in my health.

WHEN LIFE INTERVENES

Those whose steps are guided by the LORD,
whose way God approves,
may stumble, but they will never fall,
for the LORD holds their hand.
—*Psalm 37:23–24, New American Bible*

Weddings. Funerals. A child's broken arm. A tax audit. A leaky roof. A fender bender. A friend in crisis. A sudden windfall . . .

Even if you suffer from serious illness, life intervenes, interrupts your daily routine, wrenches you from one track to another, and forces your attention from your regular activities to wonderful events, terrible crises . . . Life's stumbling blocks.

We cannot avoid life's interventions. Sometimes we cannot even prepare for them. And when we have to contend with serious health issues on top of the other events in life that demand our attention, we can quickly feel overwhelmed and incapable of handling it all. Like a boat in choppy water, we can be thrown this way and that.

Sometimes we might feel as if we are dangerously close to being dashed on the jagged rocks of the shoreline.

If we allow life's events to take hold of us and shake us up, we will certainly be lost. We will lose sight of what we need to do to stay healthy, possibly even stopping our medical treatment because we "don't have the time." We could become so engrossed in others' problems that we don't take the time to solve our own. We might become so busy that we forget to pray, or we're so tired by the end of the day that we don't have the energy.

Letting life grab hold of us can take us farther from our spiritual center and make us more vulnerable to harm. By twisting and turning us, it can make us so unsteady that we become open to spiritual attack. By thinking we have to handle all of life's "curveballs" ourselves, we can forget that God is there to help us, that in fact we *need* God more than ever.

Every day it is important to keep an active prayer life moving, growing, and deepening. We never know when the next surprise will befall us, when the next time will be that our attention will be pulled from our routine to something urgent, but God certainly knows.

His support during the "calm" times is tinged with his knowledge that we will be tested and challenged.

His grace, which flows to us at all times, is a kind of armor against the times when our lives will be turned upside down— what a wonderful thing that is!

Focusing on the Lord takes practice. So, too, does the act of lifting up to him our troubles *and not taking them back again*. The more that prayer and reflection are a part of our daily lives, the more we will have a reservoir of faith and prayer "stored up" in preparation for the difficulties life brings.

The assurance in the above reading from Psalms cannot be understated. If our steps are "guided by the Lord" and if our way is approved by him, we might stumble but we will never fall.

We might have problems, we might be challenged, but our boat will never be dashed upon the rocks. Rather, God will steer us to safety. This is a great comfort, especially with all we have to deal with in terms of our health and "regular" lives.

Even good surprises require extra attention and cause stress; knowing that God is "holding our hands" gives us hope that no matter the life event, we will not fall apart.

The next time life intervenes in your world, take a deep breath.

Lift up a prayer to the Lord.

Ask for his guidance and support.

Know that God will be with you.

And he will never let you fall.

*O Lord, I can be so scattered because of all the things
that life throws at me.
Help me to keep my focus on you,
so that I might lift up these events and crises and ride
through them,
still holding on to your hand,
still staying firmly on my feet.*

ADAPTING TO CHANGE

There is a time for everything,
A season for every activity under heaven.

· · ·

A time to search and a time to lose,
A time to keep and a time to throw away.
—*Ecclesiastes 3:1, 6, New Living Translation*

Just before I was diagnosed with lupus, I went on vacation to Hawaii. I love the ocean and am fascinated by all that lives beneath its salty blue waves, so I was particularly excited to go snorkeling in the ocean for the first time in my life. But, oh, that leap into the water! The thought of jumping into the sea terrified me. I was surrounded by many other people and had a life preserver. The waters looked inviting and I knew that there were wonders to be explored beneath them. But I couldn't get started. Finally I grabbed hold of the metal bar along the stairway leading off one side of the catamaran and gingerly stepped into the ocean lapping about its steps. The other snorkelers were already enjoying themselves, paddling contentedly as though born into the aquatic activity. I turned my head and looked both ways, as if to check the "traffic" on each side of me. Suddenly my hands slipped and I lost hold of the bar. My feet fell from the stairs. I was in.

I flailed about in the water for a few seconds and then curiosity overcame apprehension. As if led by a gentle, unseen hand, I righted myself, donned my snorkel gear, and dipped my face into the ocean. What an incredible sight! There were brilliantly colored tropical fish darting here and there, sea turtles gliding among them, corals creating a fantastic garden of nooks and crannies for moray eels to hide in, and a play of light from above that threw everything into a joyful, vibrant display of natural delight. I couldn't see enough. I paddled this way and that, coming up for a look around only long enough to make sure I wasn't getting too swept away. Of course, in my heart, I was. And so was my fear, my hesitation at letting myself be carried along in the warm blue Hawaiian waters. God's creation was surely never more thrilling than during that wonderful afternoon! I was the last one to go back onto the catamaran.

Four months later I was diagnosed with lupus. Along with the diagnosis came many constraints, one of which being that I have to limit my sun exposure almost completely. This was (and still is) very hard to take. I'd love to be able to see the ocean world again, to feel the buoyant water and be part of it, if only for a while. But unless there is a cure for the disease or unless the Lord chooses to cure me, I won't be able to go snorkeling, nor will I even be able to sit on the beach and behold the daylight as it tickles and teases my beloved ocean.

I mourned the loss of all sorts of things that I lost because of lupus, but especially the experience of ever again seeing firsthand the teeming life beneath the ocean. "That was then," I had to keep telling myself, many times with tears. "The Lord has other things in store for me now." I didn't know what those things were (or are); much like being poised on the edge of the catamaran, I trembled (and still do) when I thought of what the Lord might plunge me into next. But I had to trust (and I do trust) that he would be with me all along the way. Indeed, never before have I become so acutely aware of the importance of this reading from Ecclesiastes. Our lives, just like the life that grows and dies beneath the ocean's surface, always moves, always changes.

In the months and years since my diagnosis, change hasn't stopped but rather has continued with a vengeance. I'm learning to substitute activities that I can enjoy for those that I can no longer participate in. Instead of jumping into the ocean myself, I belong to the local aquarium and keep fish of my own. I find sadness at letting go of what once was, but surprising joy in the new possibilities open to me. My mourning has become dancing so very often, and my sadness has turned to renewed wonder at how incredibly the Lord works—all the time!

Above all, I realize more fully that change is, ironically, a constant in our lives. It is not always easy. It is sometimes very painful. But it is. And so is the Lord, the gentle hand that's guiding us through every time, every season, in our many-colored lives, and bringing us through with hope, faith, and quiet, sublime happiness.

O Lord, Creator of all things,
let me have more faith, not less, as changes bring pain.
Give me creativity and strength to find ways
to witness to you
through new activities and experiences.
And let me continue to know that you have wonders
in store for me,
even if my life seems to turn upside down.

AVOIDING TOXIC RELATIONSHIPS

"And if a village won't welcome you or listen to you, shake off its dust from your feet as you leave. It is a sign that you have abandoned that village to its fate."

—*Mark 6:11, New Living Translation*

I interviewed a rabbi once, a Jewish chaplain at a very large medical center. He has made it his life's work to reflect upon and study the relationship between healing and spirituality. During the course of our talk, he said, "You wouldn't think of drinking poison or putting something toxic into your body. Why should you think of bringing toxic people into your life?"

This question has stayed with me ever since. Why *do* we allow toxic individuals to have a place in our lives? Is it because we as Christians feel we should not "preach only to the converted"? Is it because we feel a deep insignificance in ourselves and don't feel worthy to "pass judgment" upon others?

In Mark's gospel, Jesus' message seems very clear. "If a village won't welcome you or listen to you, shake off its dust from your feet as you leave." To me, that says don't spend a lot of time with people who shun you or turn a deaf ear to what you say. But as much as Jesus gave us this message, he also gave us the example of associating with prostitutes, tax collectors, and other "unsavory" characters in his society.

What is the difference between what Jesus did and what he said? What significance does this have for our lives?

Jesus was always ready to forgive people's sins. He also commanded them to "sin no more." His message in Mark contains the follow-through to these actions: if a village or people didn't accept his Word, then the disciples were expected to leave.

As we strive to create healthful environments for ourselves, we need to be true to our Christian calling. Of course, we need to bring God's message of salvation to as many people as we can. This means witnessing to nonbelievers, and it means associating with them to a certain extent. But if people turn on us or try to bring unhealthful attitudes or beliefs into our lives, we have to do what is necessary to move away from them. Sometimes this is not easy, especially if we are in partnership with the "toxic person" in question. Always we have to keep our focus on God's goodness and mercy. But we should not sacrifice ourselves or our health because others insist upon it or drive us to it.

I like the image painted by the rabbi of not ingesting poison into the body and not bringing toxic people into my life. As I've moved along in my new life with lupus, I've been very conscious of carefully assessing my relationship with others to make sure that they are healthy ones. Where relationships have fallen away or become unhealthful, I've prayed, witnessed, and sometimes taken measures to separate myself out of them. Where God has revealed the need to make repairs or changes, I've tried to do that, too.

Changes are inevitable in anyone's life. Relationships, too, go through an ebb and flow. Sometimes they become damaging to our well-being.

As you progress in your prayer life and center yourself

more firmly upon God's will for you, you will have an easier time discerning which relationships are beneficial for you and which are toxic. You will also be given the wisdom to know how to handle those toxicities so that you protect yourself and stay on track with God. In doing this, you will reach even higher levels of spiritual insight. Your prayer life will deepen. You will feel surrounded in soul and body with support and comfort and joy like never before.

God's hand is in all lives upon earth, the saved and the unsaved. We can be sure that he will deal with us, at the end of our stay on earth, just as he will deal with those people who refuse to hear his Word. So we can leave the battle to the Lord, and the final judgment, too, and carry on in our lives in a way that is nurturing and holy and as devoid as possible of any poisons in our bodies and our souls.

Heavenly Father, I sometimes get into relationships
that are not good for me.
Please help me better discern how I relate to
the people in my life
and give me the wisdom to know when a relationship
is not giving you glory and is harmful to me.
Bring me courage to avoid toxic relationships
and help nurture what is good and just in all things.

GOD'S LOVE FOR US

> For I am convinced that neither death, nor life, nor angels, nor prin-
> cipalities, nor present things, nor future things, nor powers, nor
> height, nor depth, nor any other creatures will be able to separate us
> from the love of God in Christ Jesus our Lord.
>
> —*Romans 8:38–39, New American Bible*

How reassuring this reading from Romans is!
Each day we face pressures and temptations that could
easily steer us away from our godly paths. We stumble, we
doubt, we do things that we wish we hadn't. Yet through all
of this and more, God's love for us is assured through Christ
Jesus our Lord.

I know of no other being whose love is so assured. In our
society, fads come and go. People change jobs, moving from
one beloved career to another. Friends, too, can be temporary
and, sadly, even some marriages fail.

Only God loves us so completely that nothing will sway
him or move him otherwise.

So, how do we treat God?

If someone close to us loves us, we tend to be very appre-
ciative. We probably want to love that person back and do
things that demonstrate how we feel. We apologize if we of-
fend our loved one, and we feel horrible if we miss a birthday,
anniversary, or other milestone.

If we love a particular collectible or career, we strive to learn all about it and invest time and money into really diving into its "world." If we love where we live, we take great pains to maintain and beautify it.

If we love a pet, don't we pamper it? If we love a car, don't we take care of it well? If we have a favorite pair of shoes, don't we make sure they don't get scuffed?

If we love God . . . ?

In my humanness, with all of my failings, I cannot imagine being as loving as God. Oh, I want to be! But my life is such that it works against being consistent in my other relationships, so I'm naturally fearful about failing when it comes to God. My illness often renders me unreliable. I find that as I develop more and different symptoms, I change my activities, likes and dislikes, accordingly. As I've grown in spirit and through trials, I've even evolved out of friendships and other relationships.

There are forces at work in the world to draw me away from God, too. And although I combat them as best I can, sometimes in my weakness I fall short.

But even as I write this, I know he knows me from failings to achievements. He knows that I *want* to love him all the time, although sometimes I don't necessarily demonstrate it. And he loves me all the same.

How wonderful is that? How awesome?

How remarkable that One as all-powerful and all-knowing as God would love me and you so completely and forever.

Another amazing aspect of this reading from Romans is that Paul doesn't just *believe* in God's forever love, he is *convinced* of it. And in that, I am in complete accord. When I think of all the ways God has worked in my life to protect me, comfort me, and bring me closer to him, I cannot help but be convinced, too, that he must love me entirely, even when I don't fully comprehend why or how.

We cannot fully understand God.

We cannot completely know him, for he is all.

But we can rest in the truth that, as long as we believe and reach for a life of holiness through our Lord Jesus Christ, he loves us.

No matter what.

O my Lord, your love for me fills my heart with joy
and my eyes with wonder.
I cannot stop praising you for such a wondrous gift!
Please help me to live worthy of your love
and resist all things that would tear me away from you.

THE PRAYING SPIRIT

"But when you pray, go to your inner room, close the door, and pray to your Father in secret. And your Father, who sees in secret, will repay you. In prayer, do not babble like the pagans, who think they will be heard because of their many words. Do not be like them. Your Father knows what you need before you ask him."

—*Matthew 6:6–8, New American Bible*

A quiet place.
A holy place.
A ready heart.
An open mind.

These are the things that we need in order to have a true praying spirit.

We do not need to wail and moan. We do not need to speak volumes of well-crafted words. We have only to present ourselves, broken as we are, and reach out to the Lord to fix us.

There is, of course, a time for community prayer and praise. There is a time to raise the roof with song.

But all praise, all song, begins with the quiet kernel of thought and reflection. And that is what we need to strive for as we deepen our personal life with the Lord.

As we see in this reading from Matthew, God "knows what [we] need before [we] ask him." But how many of us still insist upon giving God a laundry list of requests each time we sit down to pray? Or how often do we wait until we can assume the "perfect" prayer position before we start in?

The praying spirit does not call for a litany of intercessions, and we don't always need to be on our knees to approach the Lord in prayer. We don't have to be in the same room each time we pray, either. Our "quiet place" can be in the middle of a traffic jam or in the small corner of our room. We can lift up our hearts while changing a diaper. We can bring God to our place of employment. We make our praying place holy by the way in which we approach communicating with God. We communicate with him most perfectly when we empty ourselves of ourselves and allow him to enter our hearts and souls fully, completely.

If you embrace the full meaning of having a "praying spirit," you might find that the idea of "prayer time" is replaced by a more all-encompassing sense of constant connection with God. If you adopt a willingness to listen to him everywhere, all ways, you will hear him as you drive to the soccer game, tuck your children in for the night, and wash the evening dishes. You will find that you need to say less and you will listen more. Your heart will be so filled as to overflow with love for God.

You will never be alone.

A friend of mine once spoke enthusiastically about the man she was dating. "We don't even have to say anything to each other. It's like we're communicating all the time, even when we don't talk!"

This is the kind of relationship with the Lord that can transcend our humanness and bring us more fully into a holiness with God.

I do not shy away from prayer with others, but sometimes even in the midst of community prayer, I find myself falling silent. Because of their intrinsic limitations, words cannot plumb the depths of my love for God, nor can they fully express all that I hope for and want to strive for in him. Even the silent parts of a religious service can have a deeper meaning than the spoken ones—all because the Spirit is allowed to move without restraint from people's words and requests.

As you adopt a truly faithful praying spirit, you will find wonders and joy that you never knew. And you will crave more quiet time with the Lord, even in the midst of a busy day.

Yes, less talk and more prayer truly bring calm and peace—gifts that we do not have enough of in our challenged lives.

O Lord, give me a true praying spirit.
Let me not boast of my supplication,
but approach you humbly and quietly
so that I may hear your voice and feel your spirit
filling me with more faith and wisdom.

A New and Glorious Day

*And we have the word of the prophets made more certain, and you
will do well to pay attention to it, as to a light shining in a dark place,
until the day dawns and the morning star rises in your hearts.*
—*2 Peter 1:19, New International Version*

Remember when you first believed? What a new and glorious day that was! Nothing, not even the most mundane item in your kitchen cupboard, looked the same. Since that time you have been tested in fire and given many challenges. Your health has suffered greatly, and at times you have been sorely tempted to give up. But when you passed through that night of unbelief, you awakened to a new self. And nothing *will* ever be the same.

The same brightness and hope, the same childlike wonder is with you now, although you might not feel it. As you move ahead in your Christian walk, and illness comes upon you bringing pain, you might find yourself getting away from the feelings you had when you first accepted Christ. You might not be able to get in touch with that spark of newness and surrender that brought you to your knees at the feet of Our Savior.

But that spark still burns within you. And it can kindle your heart with warmth and comfort, even in the midst of your most horrible day.

To arrive back where you began, retrace your steps. Remember what it was like before you accepted Christ. How did you feel? How did you act? How deep was the emptiness inside of you? How great was the self-doubt?

Bring yourself forward into the moments before your great surrender to the Lord. What moved you? What exploded in your heart? How clearly did you see? How sharply did you feel?

Now, walk through the first hours and days of your conversion. What was different than before? How did others react to you? What did you like most about yourself? How hungry were you for the Word of God and for teaching that could bring you more knowledge about your new life in Christ?

Stop a moment. Breathe. Let these early feelings wash over you like a cleansing rain. Let them take away the layers of trial and error that have happened since you surrendered to our Lord. Let them make you shining and new again, like the young child of God that you were.

Take some time to think of ways that you can keep your early enthusiasm and strength for our Lord alive in your current hours and days. Remember that there is nothing wrong with being joyful in the spirit, and there is nothing wrong with being childlike in trust and faith in God. We don't have to be ashamed to be hungry for the Word, nor do we have to make excuses for wanting to learn as much as we can about that in which we believe. In fact, our Lord *wants* us to be as "little children." He *desires* us to be alive in him. He *loves* us to seek greater knowledge and understanding.

If you cannot quite get through your inhibitions to recapture your early feelings of belief in Christ, read. Read Scripture. Let the words of the Old Testament and the New come to you and show you how early prophecies were made real in the person of Jesus Christ. Find the spark of your new faith there, among the tales of God's power and salvation. Let your eyes and heart be filled with how God is all, over all.

Each day we live will bring new struggles. We will constantly be challenged to keep our spirits fresh and our faith whole. Sometimes it will seem as if we are moving through a dark tunnel or an ebony night, where our souls are tired. But be assured, the word of the prophets has been fulfilled. Jesus Christ is Lord.

The morning star will rise again in your heart!

You will walk through darkness to a new and glorious day.

O my Lord, sometimes I am so tired and feel so old.
Help me recapture my early enthusiasm for you
and my hunger for your Word and wisdom.
Let me remember how wonderful it was to accept you
and bring you back in to my life again and again
so that I may always be moving ahead
into a new and glorious day.

You Have Already Won!

"For God so loved the world that he gave his one and only Son, that whoever believes in him shall not perish, but have eternal life. For God did not send his Son into the world to condemn the world, but to save the world through him."

—*John 3:16–17, New International Version*

Not long ago, the gospel choir that I conducted for thirteen years seemed very low in energy. We'd just been through a long season of rehearsals and services, but in the past, those things had revved us up, not brought us down. In the middle of one particularly "blah" rehearsal, it occurred to me that a bit of positive visualization might help.

"Okay, now I want you to sing this piece as if you've won the lottery," I told them.

"The lottery?" some asked, obviously wondering what place this concept had in a Christian setting.

"The *spiritual* lottery," I clarified my thoughts. "In fact, we don't think about this very often, but we have *already* won!"

What a difference this idea made in the way the singers attacked their parts. The song crackled with energy and enthusiasm. I could envision the people in our congregation on their feet with the joy that the song held, and with the hope, too. I myself was swept away with the spirit.

In other parts of my life, the reality of my salvation through our Lord Jesus Christ makes me happier than I would be if I'd won the multimillion-dollar, multistate megalottery! For God's promise holds not fleeting monetary gain, but spiritual lifting, an eternity with him, a heaven unimaginable in majesty.

That God "so loved the world that he gave his one and only Son" is such a powerful testimony to our value to the Lord—a value beyond compare. How mightily humble it makes me feel . . . and how overjoyed! Truly, when I think of it, I am like the person jumping up and down with unbridled joy . . . except my joy is forever.

Through your faith in the Lord and through your life of godliness, you too have *already* won. There is no need to wonder and wait, no need to tremble with anticipation. There is no chance that your "numbers" will not be chosen, no possibility that something will go wrong. God loves you. He has *saved* you.

In sickness or in health, your life is made whole through your faith and through the Salvation of our Lord. Whether you feel physical pain or not, you know that your place is assured in heaven. It is a beautiful place, with no pain and endless time to offer thanks to our God in praise.

Let your happiness and gratitude, your joy and energy, burst forth from you in every song, in every way.

Turn your weeping into laughter and your sorrow into dance.

Feel the presence of God that is uniquely yours.

Tell others of the glory that can be theirs.

This life of illness can be very hard. But I cannot imagine what it would be like without the Lord in my life. He is the richest blessing, the most valuable gift I could ever receive. May your life, too, be filled with him. May you feel the tenderness and care, the strength and power of all that he is and can do.

And may you sing a rousing song of gladness, loud enough to wake the most skeptical listener, as you witness to the bounty of God.

I . . . You . . . *We* have already won!

O my God, thank you!
Let me always remember to sing your praises
in whatever I do or say.
Give me more grace and fire to ignite the flame of your
spirit in others.
And let me not be of this world,
but only of your world,
all of my days.

SOURCES

ABOUT THE AUTHOR

Maureen Pratt is an ambassador for the Arthritis Foundation and works closely with other health-related organizations, including the Lupus Foundation of America. Ms. Pratt is a popular speaker on lupus, chronic illness, and meditation and prayer. As a lupus patient, she advocates for research and treatment of this disease that affects approximately 2 million people in the United States. She is coauthor of *Taking Charge of Lupus: How to Manage the Disease and Make the Most of Your Life* and author of *The First Year—Hypothyroidism: An Essential Guide for the Newly Diagnosed.*

Ms. Pratt can be reached at www.maureenpratt.com